GOOD SUGAR,
BAD SUGAR

GOOD SUGAR, BAD SUGAR

How to Power Your Body and Brain with Healthy Energy

CHRISTOPHER VASEY, N.D.

Translated by Jon E. Graham

Healing Arts Press
Rochester, Vermont

Healing Arts Press
One Park Street
Rochester, Vermont 05767
www.HealingArtsPress.com

SUSTAINABLE **Certified Sourcing**
FORESTRY
INITIATIVE www.sfiprogram.org
SFI-00854

Text stock is SFI certified

Healing Arts Press is a division of Inner Traditions International

Originally published in French under the title *Sucre et santé: Distinguer les bons des mauvais sucres* by Éditions Jouvence, www.editions-jouvence.com, info@editions-jouvence.com
First U.S. edition published in 2020 by Healing Arts Press

Note to the reader: This book is intended as an informational guide. The remedies, approaches, and techniques described herein are meant to supplement, and not to be a substitute for, professional medical care or treatment. They should not be used to treat a serious ailment without prior consultation with a qualified health care professional.

Cataloging-in-Publication Data for this title is available from the Library of Congress

ISBN 978-1-62055-808-9 (print)
ISBN 978-1-62055-809-6 (ebook)

Printed and bound in the United States by Lake Book Manufacturing, Inc. The text stock is SFI certified. The Sustainable Forestry Initiative® program promotes sustainable forest management.

10 9 8 7 6 5 4 3 2 1

Text design by Virginia Scott Bowman and layout by Priscilla Baker
This book was typeset in Garamond Premier Pro with Cache, Helvetica Neue, and Avenir used as display typefaces

To send correspondence to the author of this book, mail a first-class letter to the author c/o Inner Traditions • Bear & Company, One Park Street, Rochester, VT 05767, and we will forward the communication, or contact the author directly at **www.christophervasey.ch.**

CONTENTS

Introduction   1

PART 1
. . . .
Understanding the Harmful Effects
of Bad Sugars

1 The Overconsumption of Refined Sugar:
A Brief History   4

2 The Good Sugars and the Bad Sugars:
Whole vs. Refined   20

3 Carbohydrates:
The Major Sugar Family   39

4 Blood Sugar Level:
Variations and Regulation   47

5 Diseases Caused by Bad Sugars:
From Deficiencies to Diabetes   57

6 Reactive Hypoglycemia:
Body Disturbances and Sugar Dependency   72

7 Test Yourself for Reactive Hypoglycemia:
Diet and Symptoms Questionnaires   87

8 The Glycemic Index:
Food Rankings and Their Effect on Blood Sugar Levels   92

PART 2
....
A Practical Guide to Replacing Bad Sugars
with Good Sugars

9 Identifying and Eliminating Bad Sugars   108

10 Eating Good Sugars—
Options and Replacements   122

11 Eating Enough Slow Sugars   132

12 Adding Proteins to Extend
the Glycemic Curve   137

13 Making Breakfast a Priority   144

14 Evaluating Other Causes of
Energy Depletion and Sugar Cravings   150

Conclusion   160

Bibliography   162

Index   163

INTRODUCTION

Sugar is one of the most valuable nutritive substances for the human body, as it supplies the body with the fuel it needs to function properly. Every motor requires a specific fuel in order to run: gas or electricity for automobiles, electricity for the vacuum cleaner, coal for a steam locomotive, and so on. Our "organic motor"—our physical body—is no exception to this rule, and its fuel is sugar. When it is burned in the cells, sugar provides the body with the essential energy it needs to successfully carry out its various tasks.

Sugar is, therefore, beneficial for the body. But we often hear of its many harmful effects: it attacks tooth enamel and causes cavities, it leads to weight gain, it causes diabetes, and so on.

How can a substance be both beneficial and harmful at the same time? In fact, there are good and bad forms of sugar. The good sugars are the ones offered by nature in the forms of fruit, honey, grains, and potatoes. The bad sugars are those that are man-made. These include refined white sugar; refined starches, such as all-purpose flour, that convert to sugar in the body; and all the food products that are based on them: candies, soft drinks, chocolate, white bread, white-flour pasta, and so on.

People in the Western world consume vast quantities of bad sugars. As a result, there are numerous health problems, yet

1

unaware of the source of their problems, the unwell and the sick continue to ingest the very sugars that caused their health to decline.

The purpose of this book is to show how these bad sugars have invaded our diet and jeopardized our health, and to offer guidelines for diet correction or improvement. It will explain how to get rid of the bad sugars and what to replace them with, and where to find the good sugars. It will also discuss how to reduce cravings for sweets and ensure optimum results in the body's production of energy.

All these measures are intended to allow readers to protect themselves against diseases and disorders created by sugar and show them how to take full advantage of a higher level of energy—one that will engender enthusiasm and joy in life.

PART 1

Understanding the Harmful Effects of Bad Sugars

For hundreds of thousands of years, human beings have eaten the sugars that nature has provided to them. But over the past two hundred years, humans have been primarily consuming the refined white sugar they manufacture themselves. It just so happens that this sugar causes many of the illnesses that afflict the modern individual. This refined sugar is difficult to metabolize correctly—especially when eaten in large quantities, as is currently the case—because it is not in tune with human physiology. Nature never foresaw that our bodies would be using a sugar like this.

THE OVERCONSUMPTION OF REFINED SUGAR

A Brief History

Refined white sugar looks like a real food, but it is not really food. It is what we call a fake food.

FAKE FOODS

Fake foods are edible items that have been produced by humans. They do not have the same characteristics as the true foods that are offered to us by nature, which all consist of a number of different nutrients. Fake foods consist of only an extremely limited number of nutrients, and these are present in amounts that are too little or too great to be effective.

These foods are manufactured using food extracts, which are found in a concentrated form in the fake food. For example, white sugar from sugar beets, refined flour from the starch of grains, and lard from pig fat. Among the fake foods that have a refined sugar base we find white table sugar, candy, jams and jellies, syrups, soft drinks, pastries, and so on, among the myriad other sweets that have been invented by human beings.

The term *fake* comes from the fact that these so-called foods have almost no nutritional value, and thus are really not fit for consumption as part of a healthy diet. In any case, they are not suitable as substitutes for a real food item in a regular diet because they are not beneficial for the body. They are, to the contrary, quite harmful to physical health. They have a high calorie count but are extremely low in vitamins, minerals, and so on, and their often-abundant calories are empty calories. Their sole contribution is energy without any of the valuable nutrients the body needs, and which can be found in all the foods that nature provides.

🖐 Good to Know

The purpose behind the manufacture of fake foods is not to contribute to the health of the people who consume them but is entirely commercial for profit. For example, refined sugar is easy to produce in large quantities at a low price. Its white color makes it attractive, it keeps well, and it has a flavor that answers the desires of the consumer.

REFINED SUGAR: A SUPERCONCENTRATED PRODUCT

Refined sugar is a fake food composed of 99.6 percent sucrose. No real food provided by nature has such a high concentration of solids. Even foods that have the highest contents of dry matter, such as beans and other leguminous plants, still contain around 10 percent water. Refined sugar, in contrast, has only 0.4 percent water content. Furthermore, the solid materials of real food, its components, are of different types. Soy, for example, contains 29.9 percent carbohydrates, 18.1 percent lipids, 35 percent proteins, 5 percent cellulose, and 3.3 percent minerals and vitamins. Refined white sugar, meanwhile, contains only one single component: sugar in the form of sucrose (with several extremely insignificant traces of minerals).

Honey, which is the sweetest natural food, has a 77.2 percent sugar content. Honey is a food that can be consumed only in modest amounts, however, because nature offers limited quantities of it. The complete opposite is true of white sugar, which is available in abundant quantities.

Among the other sugary foods provided by nature, fresh fruits contain an average sugar content of around 12 percent, with the lowest content found in strawberries (7.7 percent) and the highest content found in figs and grapes (16.6 percent). Dried fruits obviously contain a noticeably higher sugar content because fresh fruits become more concentrated when their water content is removed. The average sugar content of dried fruits is more than 60 percent. The sugar content for dried pears is 62.5 percent, while that of dried prunes and raisins is about 69.7 percent.

Sweet vegetables have a much lower sugar content than fruits. Red beets and carrots have around 8.4 percent while the sugar content of a raw onion is about 9.8 percent. One exception is the sweet potato; its sugar content is 26 percent.

> Although many foods provided by nature contain sugar, they all have other components and none are as concentrated as white sugar.

WHITE SUGAR IS DIFFICULT TO METABOLIZE

Because nature has never made any allowances for white sugar being introduced into the human body, our bodies perceive this substance as foreign and dangerous. When high quantities of sugar are consumed, the body immediately reacts with signs of aggression and intolerance. This is not something that happens with normal foods. This is why volunteers who ingested 150 grams of white sugar at one time during experiments experienced accelerated pulse rate, rising blood pressure, and flushed faces. Their urine contained sugar (glycosuria), which is normally not the case. This defensive reaction only occurred because it was white sugar. Such a response does not take place at all following consumption of unrefined sugars.

During a grape cure, a diet originally developed in the 1920s to treat cancer, patients can consume almost five pounds of grapes a day—twice the 150 gram-dose used in the above experiment—without any glycosuria or defensive reactions appearing, because grapes are a food found in nature.

The distinction between good and bad sugars is, we can see, no fantasy. White sugar is a bad sugar, a fake food.

TOO LARGE A PLACE IN THE DIET

Unfortunately, fake food white sugar is not eaten only in small quantities from time to time but is ingested regularly in large amounts.

Although the amount of consumption per person and per country varies from one study to the next, it is generally agreed that daily consumption of white sugar in European countries is around 100 grams, or 3.5 ounces, which translates to 44 average-sized sugar cubes, or 21 teaspoons. In the United States, the most recent data from 2017 shows 126 grams, or 27 teaspoons, per day on average. These sugar totals include not only sweetener the consumer personally adds to food and drinks but also sugar that has been added to improve the flavor of all kinds of packaged foods that are sold commercially.

These figures represent the average individual consumption in a country. All of the country's inhabitants are included in the calculation, including infants, toddlers, and the very old, who usually do not consume as much sugar. This calculation also includes all those in the broader population who consume no or very little sugar, in most cases because they are aware of its adverse effects. This means that a substantial portion of the population is eating far more than 126 grams of sugar a day, perhaps even 200 grams! The top 10 percent of sugar consumers get as much as 40 percent of their daily calories from sugar.

Instead of presenting the rate of white sugar consumption on a daily basis, we can look at this consumption annually. An individual who is consuming 126 grams of sugar a day is taking in 46 kilograms (approximately 101 pounds) a year, and the annual rate leaps up to 73 kilograms (161 pounds) for someone eating 200 grams of white sugar a day. For many adults this consumption is greater than their own body weight.

POUNDS OF FOOD THE AVERAGE AMERICAN CONSUMES IN ONE YEAR

Milk and non-cheese dairy products	600
Fruit	273
Vegetables (except corn and potatoes)	217
Corn and potatoes	198
Wheat flour and foods made from grains	192
Meat	184
Sugar	152
Fats and oils	86
Eggs	32
Cheese	31
Coffee and chocolate	21
Fish and shellfish	16
Tree nuts and peanuts	12
Beans	7

Source: Compiled by Visual Economics, USDA, and industry-specific sites.

To get a good sense of how large consumption of white sugar actually is, we need to compare it with other foods we eat on a regular basis.

The table on page 8 from a 2016 study shows the consumption of different kinds of foods per person. The foods have been listed in decreasing order of quantities consumed.

This table shows that in 2016 American consumption of white sugar was equal to 56 percent of that of fruits, 70 percent of that of vegetables, and 800 percent more than nuts and beans.

The comparisons in this chart are only between the foods themselves. However, real foods do not consist solely of sugar. Fruits contain an average of 20 percent sugar while foods made from grains have around 50 percent. What these percentages represent for the year are an actual intake of 54 pounds of sugar from fruits and 96 pounds from grain products. If we compare these figures with the consumption rate of 152 pounds of white sugar, we see that the average American citizen is consuming three times as much white sugar as sugar coming from fruits. It is quite clear, therefore, that the place occupied by sugar in our diet is enormous! The situation is the same in Canada, Europe, and most industrialized countries.

HOW DID WHITE SUGAR INVADE OUR DIET?

White sugar holds a prominent place in our daily diet. How did we ever reach this state? History offers two factors that explain how this invasion took place:

- The expansion of sugarcane cultivation, which started as a very regional practice and eventually spread all around the world, traveling from Indonesia (where it originated) into

Asia, then into southern Europe, and finally the Americas.

■ The increased perfection of farming and refining methods, which made it possible to transform this rare and expensive product into one that is cheap and abundant, and therefore accessible to everyone.

These two factors, however, were only able to exercise such influence by virtue of a third factor that is physiological in nature: the body's need for sugar in order to function properly and the innate appeal of this fuel to human beings, an attraction that is materialized in the desire and pleasure of eating sweet foods.

Let's now take a quick look at just how, historically speaking, this invasion unfolded.

📖 A Little History

A native of the islands of the South Pacific, the sugarcane plant can grow as high as sixteen feet. It resembles bamboo with its long oval stalk that is interspersed every eleven to twelve inches by knots, from which sprout long, slender leaves. But in contrast to bamboo, the stalk of the sugarcane is extremely high in sugar: 15 to 25 percent of its weight consists of sucrose.

The first domesticated sugar crop was sugarcane, believed to have been developed from wild varieties growing in the East Indies, probably New Guinea, around 8000 BCE. At that time usage primarily consisted of sucking the ends of sugarcane stalks to enjoy their flavor or chewing them in order to extract their sugary sap.

It was around 1000 BCE when sugarcane was introduced into India, thanks to maritime trade. This is when farming of sugarcane truly began to develop and the first techniques for extracting its sap were perfected. This made it possible to produce a beverage that was enjoyable or to blend it in culinary preparations. Because it was so high in sugar, this liquid fermented rapidly. The problem of conserving it therefore quickly became an issue. To remedy this situation the juice was exposed to sunlight on flat surfaces so that its liquid would evaporate. The sugar contained in the sap crystallized, providing a stable product. This residue was dry and brittle, similar to sand or gravel. In Sanskrit the word for both sand and gravel is *sharka*. This name was then used to designate sugar. It is the origin of the English word *sugar* as well as the French word *sucre*.

Knowledge of the gustatory virtues of sugarcane and the possibility of obtaining crystallized sugar from its stalks did not remain confined to India but made its way to the Greek world. When Alexander the Great conquered India in 325 BCE, he discovered there "the reed that gives honey without the help of bees." The Greek historian and geographer Megasthenes (born around 340 BCE) spent ten years in India and told his contemporaries about sugar on his return to Greece. This did not inspire the Greeks to cultivate sugarcane, but they did begin importing it in small quantities.

The Greek physician and botanist Dioscorides (46–90 CE) wrote the following about sugar: "There is a kind of dry honey known as sugar. Its consistency is reminiscent of salt and it crunches under the teeth."

It will be noted here that sugar is once again compared to honey. At that time honey was the best-known food with a high concentration of sugar and therefore naturally was used as a reference.

By the fourth century CE, India, which had been cultivating sugar for hundreds of years, had become expert in the art of making sugar. Documents offer evidence that by the year 350 CE, during the Gupta Dynasty, procedures for extracting and crystallizing the sap had evolved. For example, in order to extract the liquid, the sap was not simply exposed to the sun, but cooked.

In the sixth century, sugarcane cultivation made its way to China. The Chinese emperor Taizong of the Tang Dynasty (598–649 CE) took a great interest in it. He sent emissaries to India to learn their farming and extraction methods, and implemented projects to establish sugar plantations in China.

One other people of this time also took advantage of Indian expertise: the Persians. After encountering sugar during an expedition into India, they brought plants back to their native land and began growing them extensively. Over time they perfected production procedures by refining the sugar over successive cooking sessions of the sap and clarifying (purifying) the resulting syrup. Another Persian innovation was the packaging of the finished product in the form of a loaf of sugar. Because this sugar loaf was quite hard, it was given the name of "stone honey," and although it was used to some extent in cooking, its use was primarily medical. All kinds of surprising virtues were attributed to it: it was deemed to be a miraculous remedy against epidemics, and it could be used to treat the stomach, intestines, and kidneys.

During the following century (the seventh century), the Arabs invaded Persia and returned home with the secrets of sugar production. For example, sugarcane cultivation requires large amounts of water, so they developed new farming procedures with the installation of canals, to artificially irrigate the plantations. They also discovered the means for making sugar soft; because it was crystallized it had always been hard until this time. The sweet, soft balls of sugar they obtained with their methods they called *kurat al milb,* a name from which the word *caramel* has been derived.

Thanks to Arab expansion during the ninth and tenth centuries, the production and farming of sugar spread to many of the countries bordering the Mediterranean Sea: Palestine, Syria, Egypt, Cyprus, Sicily, and Spain. The sugar the Arabs produced in these regions was exported to Europe. However, sugar remained a rare and expensive commodity available to only a few of the privileged.

Sugar's renown increased in Europe during the period spanning the eleventh through thirteenth centuries, thanks to the Crusades. Crusaders included all social classes of the population, and both men and women. During their expeditions and sojourns in the Middle East, they became familiar with and learned to appreciate the various sweet preparations (caramel, pastries) prepared by the Arabs. When they returned home, they shared what they had learned about this "sugary salt."

During the thirteenth century, the Dutch and the Venetians held a monopoly on the sugar sold in Europe. Sugar consumption in the West began gradually increasing, but only among the leisure classes of society. It was during this time that the word *candy* first appeared in England. These sweets were manufactured by dipping a thread into a syrup that was oversaturated with sugar. The syrup would then crystallize along the string to form what we now call "rock candy." More than just a sweet treat, rock candy was considered to be a soothing sore throat remedy.

At the end of the fourteenth century the Spanish and the Portuguese became large sugar producers. The recently discovered lands of Central and South America offered not only large tracts of land but also a climate favorable to this kind of agriculture. There was increasing demand for new plantations, because sugarcane farming is extremely demanding and quickly depletes the soil. In consequence, sugarcane plantations multiplied throughout the New World, not only in the Spanish and Portuguese colonies, but also in those of the French and English.

This required an ever-increasing number of manual laborers, but the local pool of workers was not very numerous and refused to perform the extremely tedious labor of the plantations and sugar refineries. This was the catalyst for the capture and enslavement of thousands of Africans who were exploited to work in the sugarcane plantations (as well as cotton plantations) of the New World.

This cheap slave labor brought about a reduction in production costs, which in turn led to a drop in the price of sugar, making it accessible to other classes of society. Nonetheless, it was still costly and sugar remained a luxury product even for those who could afford to consume it. It remained as such for a long time.

📖 A Little History

In sixteenth-century France, sugar was kept under lock and key. The head of the household held the access key and monitored how much sugar could be consumed, by whom, and when.

The number of consumers and the quantities of sugar available increased constantly during the eighteenth century. The figures are highly revealing. Between 1700 and 1709 in England, the annual consumption of sugar per inhabitant was 2 kilos (4.4 lbs.). In 1800, nearly a century later, consumption had risen to 8 kilos (17.6 lbs.); in other words, four times as much. In 1900, another century later, consumption had risen to 38 kilos (approximately 84 lbs.). In 1933, it had risen to 48 kilos (nearly 106 lbs.).

The growing consumption of sugar can be explained not only by the reduction in price but also by a change in dietary habits. Because sugar was now more widely available, it could factor into the composition of an increasing number of food preparations, sometimes becoming the primary ingredient. The nineteenth century saw the invention of jam and chocolate, and all kinds of candies. Stores that specialized in the sale of candies and other sweets began opening in a number of locations. Their customers consisted of many adults, of course, but also quite a few children. These latter grew accustomed to eating sugary foods and became great consumers of sweets, which were used not only as special treats and gifts but also in child rearing, as a reward or as an inducement for good behavior.

A large number of new desserts appeared, but sugar was also used in the creation of many main courses that, although salty, contained a little sugar to heighten the flavor. The coffee, tea, and cocoa trades were also growing exponentially during this era, and encouraged the increasing consumption of sugar as, generally speaking, these beverages were sweetened to make their flavor more enjoyable.

A spectacular increase in sugar consumption occurred in every level of society during the nineteenth century. The primary cause for this great leap forward was a political event: the continental blockade instituted by Napoleon in 1806. The purpose of this blockade was to weaken England by forbidding its boats access to any European ports. The consequence was that boats laden with sugar from the plantations in America could no longer deliver their cargoes, and sugar rapidly became scarce.

Confronted by the discontent of his people, who had grown accustomed to eating sugar—and Napoleon himself seems to have had a sweet tooth—a backup solution was sought. The idea of producing sugar in Europe from a local plant began to gain ground, and different types of plants were studied for this purpose. Grapes were an early experiment, because they contain 16 grams of sugar per kilo, but their sugar was hard to crystallize and the idea was abandoned. The plant selected finally was the sugar beet. The research of various chemists (Andreas Marggraf, Franz Karl Achard, and others) offered evidence of the sugar beet's potential in this regard. Its sugar—sucrose— was identical to that found in sugarcane. Furthermore, its sugar content (15 percent to 18 percent) is practically the same as that found in sugarcane (15 percent to 25 percent).

Under Napoleon's impetus, large tracts of land were converted to the cultivation of sugar beets. Intensive farming of sugar beets began in 1811 and grew continuously from that time forward. This expansion was encouraged by the fact that the beets are easier to grow and work with than sugarcane, and beets are smaller (sugarcane can measure some 16–17 feet in length). Through selective breeding over time, sugar beets with higher sugar content were produced. This was followed by technical innovations that facilitated the extraction, decanting, and purification of the sugar. Different forms of packaging sugar were developed (more or less fine powder, granular, cubes) that also helped in making it more attractive to consumers. Larger and larger quantities of sugar were produced at lower and lower costs, and the price of sugar plummeted. Sugar was no longer a costly, rare product but had become abundant and inexpensive. Within the reach of everyone, sugar was now consumed by everyone, everywhere, in larger and larger quantities.

The consistently perfected procedures for purifying sugar finally made it possible to obtain a pristine white sugar. White sugar was born!

Today we eat sugar as if it were completely natural, but this food was completely unknown during the entire history of humanity preceding the past two centuries.

☝ **Good to Know**

Sugar production is as detrimental for the environment as it is for our bodies. Sugarcane requires massive amounts of water, and the fields are customarily torched to strip leaves, causing significant carbon emissions. Beet sugar presents a different set of problems, and 95 percent of the domestic sugar beet crop is genetically engineered.

Since the moment white sugar was "invented," its consumption has increased to the point of proven and continuous overconsumption, and refined white sugar is not what our ancestors ate. What was consumed in the past (in small quantities, moreover) was a whole food or had barely been refined; what is now consumed is stripped of any nutritive value. Human beings are overeating a product of no physiological benefit. It should therefore come as no surprise that this refined white sugar has been responsible for seriously compromising human health.

In addition to the reasons we have just looked at, the huge surge in sugar consumption during the nineteenth and twentieth centuries was also encouraged by strong support from the medical and scientific authorities of the time. They were completely hypnotized by this new man-made "food." They described it as eminently beneficial for health and general well-being. The population was encouraged to consume it in generous quantities.

One witness of this infatuation with white sugar was Dr. Paul Carton (1875–1947), a pioneer of natural medicine. In his *Traité de médicine, d'alimentation et d'hygiène naturistes* [Treatise on natural medicine, food, and health] of 1931, he described this propaganda:

If we are to take the authoritative authors at their word, sugar is a choice food that can be recommended to children and adults alike, to those enjoying good health as well as to those who are ill. They praise it in these kinds of terms: "It is the preeminent energy food. Even in the tiniest amounts, it has the highest caloric value and is the food used most quickly and completely without leaving behind any kind of digestive trace. Its dynamogenic powers are such that all it takes, when feeling fatigued, is to munch a few pieces to immediately restore your energy and feel the exhaustion dissipate. Its nutritive value is substantial. And it is so simple to use it to provide strength! It requires no culinary preparation, is easy to obtain, and is not too expensive." Here is the logical conclusion to this kind of dithyrambic presentation: "Those responsible for the management of social hygiene should offer dietary education to the masses and teach them the art of feeding themselves by making greater use of this healthy, appetizing, invigorating, and nourishing food: man-made sugar. Its already very common use must become even more widespread. It can be eaten on its own as a snack or added to other foodstuffs (oat or cornmeal, eggs, fruit), eaten also in the form of chocolate, cocoa, jams, candies, cookies, and so forth, or even dissolved in water, coffee, tea, or milk. Patients who have been losing weight can do nothing more positive than to make sugar a large part of their diet. Workers are not eating enough sugar and remain too ignorant of its many advantages. How couldn't ignorance of this nature not be harmful to laborers whose capital consists entirely of their health and vigor?" (This is the opinion of Richet, Landuzky, and others.)

This is what voices of all kinds are claiming louder and louder, and what is being printed in treatises, magazines, and newspapers. But is it true?

The answer is clearly no, so far as Dr. Carton is concerned, and he waged war against this kind of propaganda all his life. The arguments he cited are no longer in circulation today and have stopped being used, but in this earlier time they had a huge impact. Sugar consumption made its way into daily custom and became a habit that continues in full force even today.

2

THE GOOD SUGARS AND THE BAD SUGARS

Whole vs. Refined

One single word, *sugar,* is used to designate things of very different qualities. There are, in fact, good and bad sugars. From the naturopath's perspective, good sugars are the ones produced by nature, and bad sugars are the ones produced by humans. We should now take a look at which foods provided by nature answer our needs for sugar and how, by adulterating them, humans produce the bad sugars.

THE GOOD SUGARS

Nature not only "gives" us our bodies but also the foods they need to function properly. Foods are considered healthful when they are adapted to our physical organism. They are beneficial for us because they were planned for our use. Nature works on behalf of life. It does not offer foods that are harmful and destructive to the body.

Among the myriad foods that nature has put at our disposal, there are those that are rich in sugar. The sugars these foods contain are the "good sugars." They must be eaten in the form in which they are provided to us by nature, or at least one that is quite close to that form. Some transformations are therefore acceptable, such as the cooking of cereal grains, or the making of juice from whole fruit. Any change that is more drastic, such as the extraction of one of their components, should be avoided. In fact, a true food consists of a number of different parts, each one of which has an important role to play. Therefore, subtracting any of these parts should be avoided.

Some of the foods containing the good sugars offered to us by nature can be directly identified by their flavor, such as fruits, which have a sweet taste. Others do not have a sweet taste because the sugar they contain is in the form of starch.

CARBOHYDRATE FOODS WITH A SWEET TASTE

- Fresh fruits
- Dried fruits
- Fruit juices
- Sweet vegetables: carrots, beets, onions, sweet potatoes
- The juice of these vegetables and fruits
- Honey
- Whole or unrefined sugar

CARBOHYDRATE FOODS WITHOUT A SWEET TASTE

- Grains: wheat, oats, barley, and so on
- Products made from grains: bread, pasta, and so on
- Legumes: soybeans, lentils, peanuts (which, despite their name, are not a nut), and so on
- Chestnuts
- Potatoes

Note: It is understood that the fruit juices in this list have had no sugar added and that the grains are whole and unrefined.

THE BAD SUGARS

Bad sugars are obtained from the adulteration of food. This adulteration primarily consists of extracting certain components and using them separately from the rest of the food.

The most common adulteration procedures are:

- extraction of sugar
- refinement of grains

👆 Good to Know

Sugar extraction leads to the manufacture of white table sugar and confectioners' sugar. The refining of grains permits the production of all-purpose refined flour, a fake food that is just as harmful as white sugar.

The Extraction of Sugar

Although human beings have always had sweet foods such as honey and fresh fruit at their disposal, they have been attempting for a very long time to extract the sugary part from various plants so they can use it freely in a concentrated form.

Sugarcane, which contains from 15–25 percent sugar in the form of sucrose, has long been utilized for this purpose. When stalks of sugarcane are crushed and then pressed in order to extract the sugar, the only component removed from the sugarcane is water. The crystallized sugar that is produced by this procedure therefore still contains all the vitamins, minerals, and trace elements of the plant. This is whole sugar; consequently, it is considered to be a good sugar.

However, for reasons of increasing profitability, preservation, and appearance (color and texture), the sugar industry developed a more drastic method of sugar extraction.

The sap is subjected to two operations of transformation. The first is a semipurification that rids it of impurities, such as plant debris. The second transformation involves cooking the sap. The sugar contained in the sap crystallizes because of the higher temperature. The sap separates into two large parts. One of these parts remains at the top of the vat: dark molasses. This is a thick, brown residue in the form of syrup. It contains sugar but its primary characteristic is its high content of minerals, vitamins, and trace elements. The other part, a mass formed by crystallized sugar that is greater in density, is deposited on the bottom of the vat. This sugar is raw sugar. It still contains some nutrients but is no longer a whole food because it is lacking the nutrients found in the dark molasses.

The cooking procedure is repeated several times on the residual liquid obtained after each filtration of the crystallized sugar. This means that each time it is heated again, the sugar remaining in this residual liquid precipitates and produces a certain amount of crystallized sugar. Repeating the operation enables the extraction of the maximum possible quantity of sugar, but with each cooking this sugar loses more of its nutrients. Consequently it becomes a deficient sugar that falls under the heading of bad sugars.

The sugar beet contains from 15–18 percent sugar, which, like sugarcane, is also in the form of sucrose. The extraction procedures (pressure, filtration) are first and foremost the same as for sugarcane. They are followed, however, by numerous purification procedures that aim to "cleanse" the sugar to the maximum extent possible. Unfortunately this not only eliminates any plant residues but also all the vitamins and almost all of the minerals. The sugar that is obtained this way is commercially labeled "pure" because it is ostensibly the most purified, but the process has removed virtually all the nutrients other than a few minuscule traces of minerals.

In the accompanying table we can see clearly the differences between whole unrefined sugar (with blackstrap molasses), raw sugar (without blackstrap molasses but still with some nutrients), and fully refined white table sugar.

SUGAR COMPOSITION, PER 100 GRAMS: BASED ON THE RESEARCH OF DR. MAX-HENRI BÉGUIN

	WHOLE SUGAR	RAW SUGAR	WHITE SUGAR
Sucrose	74–92 g	96–97 g	99.6 g
Glucose	2–11 g	0–1 g	0 g
Fructose	3–12 g	0–1 g	0 g
Protein	0.4–1.1 g	0 g	0 g
Mineral Salts	1500–2900 mg	260–500 mg	30–50 mg
Potassium	600–1100 mg	15–150 mg	3–5 mg
Magnesium	100–180 mg	13–20 mg	0 mg
Calcium	50–170 mg	75–95 mg	10–15 mg
Phosphorus	14–80 mg	3–4 mg	0.3 mg
Iron	3–5 mg	0.5–1.3 mg	0.1 mg
Vitamins			
Provitamin A	3.9 mg	0 mg	0 mg
B_1	0.14 mg	0.01 mg	0 mg
B_2	0.14 mg	0.006 mg	0 mg
B_6	0.4 mg	0 mg	0 mg
Niacinamide	0.2 mg	0.03 mg	0 mg
B_5	1.2 mg	0.02 mg	0 mg
Vitamin C	38 mg	0 mg	0 mg

Source: Kousmine Medical Association, *La Methode Kousmine* [The Kousmine Method] (Geneva: Éditions Jouvence, 1989).

The Different Sugars

There are a number of different types of crystallized sugar sold commercially because they are produced from various stages of the refining process. For this reason it is well worth taking the trouble to introduce them and define those that are good and those that are bad.

Whole Sugar

This sugar is obtained through the evaporation of sugarcane sap. It contains all the nutrients that are found in the plant. Thus it is a good sugar. Whole sugar may be sold under the name blond, panela, rapadura, jaggery, piloncillo, muscovado, demerara, or Sucanat. Whatever the name, the label should state that the sugar is whole and unrefined.

☝ Good to Know

Partially refined sugars stand between whole sugar (which contains all the nutrients of the sugarcane) and granulated sugar (which has none left). As there are different levels of refining, there are all sorts of different kinds of partially refined sugars. The good ones are those that have been only very slightly processed and therefore are rich in vitamins and minerals. Their color is light brown to golden and they still have a slight taste of cane (blackstrap). They have not been bleached or cooked at high temperatures. If partially refined sugars have been processed too much, they become bad sugars.

Raw Sugar (Organic Sugar)

This sugar is not really raw, as it has undergone the first stage of the refining process, been heated at high temperatures, and been stripped of the nutrients contained in blackstrap molasses. It still contains traces of vitamins and minerals but far less than what can be found in whole sugar. It is therefore a bad sugar, but perhaps the least bad of the refined sugars.

Turbinado Sugar

This sugar has been only partially refined. The word *turbinado* means it has been spun in a centrifuge in the presence of steam, so that most of the outer coating of molasses is removed. It has larger crystals, but it is not a whole sugar and it belongs to the category of bad sugars.

Brown Sugar (Dark Brown, Golden Brown, Light Brown)

This can refer to sugar that is brown because it has some residual molasses content, but more commonly refers to commercial brown sugar that has up to 6.5 percent molasses added back in to refined white sugar to make it brown. In the latter case it will lose its brown color when added to hot water. In any event these are bad sugars.

Plantation Sugar

This sugar is usually found only in sugar-growing countries and is made by injecting sulfur dioxide gas into raw sugar. It belongs to the category of bad sugars.

Granulated Sugar (Table Sugar, White Sugar)

This is sugar that has been refined to the maximum extent possible. It no longer contains any nutrients. It is sold in a powdered form that has been crushed to a varying degree (fine and superfine) or in cubes. This is the preeminent form of bad sugar.

By altering granulated sugar, it is possible to obtain other kinds of sugars that are used in a variety of food preparations. All products that are based on white sugar fall under the heading of bad sugars.

Confectioners' Sugar
Ground extremely fine, this bad sugar comes in the form of a powder that is used for frosting.

Invert Sugar
This is a bad sugar that has been made soft through hydrolysis. It is used in the soft filling of candies, cookies, and pastries.

Sugar in Large Crystals
This bad sugar is used for cake and pastry decoration.

Liquid Sugar
This is white sugar that has been dissolved in water and is used to sweeten beverages, syrups, soft candies like fudge, ice cream, jams, and so forth. It is a bad sugar.

Corn Syrup
This syrup has a high glucose content; it is manufactured from corn starch. It is a bad sugar.

High-Fructose Corn Syrup
The term refers to the corn syrup described above after it has been put through a series of enzymatic processes to transform its glucose into fructose. It is a bad sugar used in a wide range of processed foods. Glucose can be used directly by almost the entire body whereas fructose must be metabolized by the liver.

Glucose Syrup (Confectioners' Syrup)
Made from the hydrolysis of starch, glucose syrup is usually made from maize, potatoes, or wheat. It is a bad sugar used to sweeten, soften, and add volume to foods.

Rock Candy

Large crystals are obtained from the slow crystallization of sugar syrup, often on a string, with coloring added. As referenced earlier, they are sold as candies and are a bad sugar.

Table Molasses

This syrup is produced from the first boiling of sugarcane or sugar syrup, and often has caramel added for color. It is a bad sugar that contains no vitamins or minerals and should not be confused with blackstrap molasses that contains all the nutrients found in sugarcane sap. Light molasses and fancy molasses are lighter versions of this type of molasses.

There are several more bad sugars that are not made from sugarcane.

Fructose

Sold as fruit sugar, it is most often extracted from corn and no longer contains any nutrients. It is sold either as a powder that has been ground more or less finely (fine or superfine) or in pieces. This is a bad sugar.

Dextrose

This substance is also sold as fruit sugar; however, its origin is one kind of starch or another. It is pure, crystallized sucrose that has been stripped of all its nutritive properties, thus a bad sugar.

Xylitol

Xylitol is an extract from the xylan of birch bark (xylan is also found in corn cobs). It has been purified; hence it has no vitamins or minerals.

Synthetic Sweeteners

Although they are not carbohydrates, we will take a brief detour to discuss these synthetic sweeteners, because they are consumed as a substitute for sugar.

A synthetic substance is one that has been created artificially in a laboratory by either copying a molecule that already exists in nature or creating a new one. In the case of sweeteners, the main characteristics of these laboratory-created molecules are sweet and very sweet. Aspartame, for example, is up to two hundred times sweeter than table sugar. But this sweetening power can be even higher: saccharine can be up to five hundred times sweeter than table sugar.

As a general rule, sweeteners are not made from sugar. Aspartame, for example, consists of two amino acids, and thus is not part of the family of carbohydrates. Because they are not sugars they do not have many of the drawbacks of sugar—dental cavities, excess weight, hyperglycemic reactions, and so forth—which is why they are often used as a substitute for granulated table sugar.

At first glance, synthetic sweeteners can appear beneficial as they make it possible to avoid the harmful effects of the bad sugars while still offering sweetness. But in reality these synthetized molecules have proven to be dangerous to the body. These are not molecules crafted by nature that can be used by the body. Because they are foreign to biological cycles and can cause a variety of health disorders, some of which are serious, their use is not at all advisable.

🖐 Good to Know

Artificial sweeteners are made in a laboratory and cannot be used by the body but can actually cause harm. Thus they should be avoided.

THE REFINEMENT OF GRAINS

Until the middle of the nineteenth century, the flour used to make bread, pasta, or crackers consisted of all the components found in the grain itself with the exception of its outer husk, which was too hard (bran). Human beings were therefore able to benefit from all the valuable nutrients offered by the grains they ground for use in their diet. Today we know this as whole grain flour. The term *whole* to designate grains was not yet used during this time because refining processes had not yet been perfected, so there was no other option.

Starting around the middle of the nineteenth century a revolution took place in the flour mills of America: traditional millstones were replaced by cylindrical metal grindstones. This was the beginning of the modern flour mill that made it easier to separate the various components of the grain and

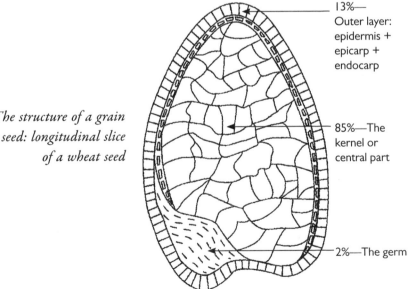

The structure of a grain seed: longitudinal slice of a wheat seed

13%—Outer layer: epidermis + epicarp + endocarp

85%—The kernel or central part

2%—The germ

obtain a lighter product that contained no germ or husk. This smoother, lighter flour gradually replaced the whole grain flour that had been used until that time. Today we call it all-purpose white flour.

From this point forward all-purpose white flour was increasingly used to make bread because it offered several advantages over its predecessor. These advantages were not dietary in nature but practical and financial. Because the flour had been stripped of its enzymes, it stayed fresh longer. It was easier to work with and provided a lighter texture. Its attractive white color was seen as a sign of refinement to the people of an era accustomed to coarser, darker bread.

? Did You Know?

All-purpose refined white flour consists exclusively of starch. It is deficient and adulterated and contains none of the vitamins, minerals, and proteins found in whole wheat flour. With all the nutrients removed it is essentially a bad sugar. Compounding the damage, it is usually bleached with either chlorine or some kind of oxide.

In order to better understand the harm refining procedures have on the quality of grains, it is helpful to know the structure of a cereal grain and the different stages of the process used to produce flour.

The Structure of a Cereal Grain

A cereal grain is composed of three major parts:

The Kernel or Central Part

This part represents 85 percent of the grain. It consists almost exclusively of starch.

The Pericarp or Husk
(Epidermis and Subcortical Layer)

This part represents 13 percent of the grain and is rich in minerals, trace elements, and vitamins. It contains barely any starch and is very high in protein.

The Germ

The germ represents a mere 2 percent of the grain but possesses an abundance of the nutrients the plant needs in order to grow.

The most valuable substances are therefore found primarily in the husk and the germ, which are in the superficial areas of the grain. The least valuable, as it is present in large amounts in nature—the starch—is found primarily in the central portion of the grain.

Production of Flour

There are three stages in the production of flour: threshing, milling, and sieving.

Threshing and Shelling

During this stage the hard and indigestible husk of the grain, which is to say the hard bran, is separated from the rest of the grain.

Milling

This operation consists of reducing the grain to a flour with the help of a millstone. Different structures of flour can be obtained depending on the type of millstone used.

- *Milling with a grindstone:* Milling was traditionally performed in gristmills using a pair of heavy millstones and powered by water or wind. The plant tissues were ripped and torn from the entire seed including all of the layers. The resulting flour particles therefore contained the nutrients belonging to several different layers of the grain. Proteins, enzymes, vitamins, and minerals were distributed throughout all the flour produced in this way. The composition of the flour particles was more homogenous, which made it difficult to separate the particles when put through a sieve to produce flour variations.

- *Milling with a cylindrical grindstone:* This is the modern system of milling. Traditional millstones have been replaced with metal cylinders, and the grains are flattened and crushed instead of torn apart. During this crushing the various layers of the grain separate from each other. The resulting flour particles no longer contain the nutrients of all of the layers but only those found in one layer. This kind of particle has a specific nutrient content that makes it easy to separate during the sieving process to produce typical kinds of flour.

Milling reduces the various parts of the grain into particles whose constitution, weight, and volume are different depending on where in the grain they originate. The smallest and finest particles are those that come from the central portion of the grain. In fact, starch is able to be ground into a much finer flour than the superficial parts of the grain, which are higher in fiber.

Sieving and Sifting

The flour that emerges in the milling process contains all the nutrients of the cereal grain. It is a whole flour and therefore a "good sugar." But flour is generally not used as it is at this stage. Two different operations are used to change its composition and thereby obtain flours of different qualities: sieving and sifting.

- *Sieving:* This operation consists of separating the bran from the flour with the help of a coarse mesh sieve. There are two kinds of bran: the large, very hard and rough bran husk, and the more tender edible bran. The harder bran is present in the complete flour but not in the whole grain flour. The latter only contains the tender bran.
- *Sifting:* The flour that has been stripped of its bran is then sifted through a series of sieves with increasingly tighter meshes. This causes the composition of the flour to change: the more of its components that are removed, the whiter it becomes and the more nutrient poor, making it a bad sugar.

The Different Types of Wheat Flour

There are literally hundreds of different types of flour, but only a few are commonly sold in American food markets. Depending on what refining processes are used during the sieving and sifting processes, the different qualities of flour are either bad or good sugars.

Whole Meal Flour (Brown, Irish-Style)

This coarsely ground flour uses all layers of the grain of white wheat, which is only superficially different from the red wheat used to produce most whole wheat flour. However, it does produce a softer flour than flour from red wheat. It contains both the hard and tender brans and is a good sugar. In the United States the internet is the best source for this type of flour.

Whole Wheat Flour

This flour, generally made from hard red wheat, is obtained by milling all parts of the grain but retaining only a small portion of the outermost layer (the tender bran). It is a good sugar.

Sprouted Wheat Flour

White wheat grains are sprouted before milling to facilitate digestion. It produces a lighter baked product but still has the nutrition of whole wheat flour. It is a good sugar.

White Whole Wheat Flour

Produced by milling hard white wheat, this flour is lighter in color and texture than flour made from red wheat but retains most of the nutrition and fiber of the wheat. Because of this we can consider it a good sugar.

Whole Wheat Pastry Flour (Light Wheat Flour)

This flour is generally made from the whole grain of soft white wheat and produces a softer, lighter-colored flour for baking. It is a good sugar.

All-Purpose Flour (White, Refined)

This flour is produced by milling the most central and lightest part of the grain kernel. It is often bleached and may include other ingredients. It is a bad sugar.

Cake Flour

This flour is highly milled and usually bleached, and while it is higher in protein than most flours, it is a bad sugar.

☝ Good to Know

Navigating the great variety of flours might be a bit confusing. Basically, the important question is whether the grains used to make the flour are *whole* or *refined*.

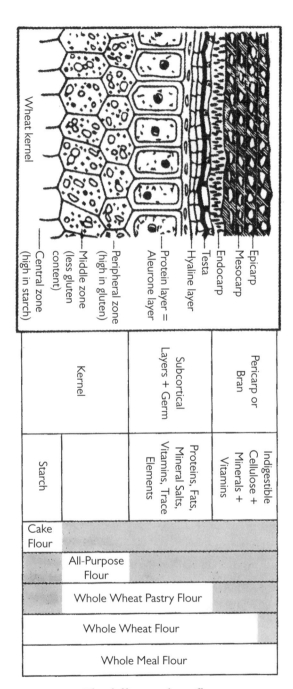

The different wheat flours

☝ Good to Know

It is often assumed that "multigrain" breads are a healthy option, but this is not necessarily the case if those grains are refined. Here again the basic question is: Is the bread made with whole or refined grains?

Other Types of Flour

Concern over gluten sensitivity has brought more flour options to U.S. markets. These are some of the most common options, usually found in natural food markets but also in some grocery stores.

Oat Flour

Made from oats rather than wheat, this flour is high in carbohydrates but is a slow, nutrient-dense source, so it is a good sugar.

Rice Flour

Rice flour, also called rice powder, is obtained by milling rice very finely. It is a good substitute for wheat flour when cooking cakes, pies, cookies, and crackers. It acts as a thickening agent and gives a crispy texture. Rice flour is a good sugar if it is made from brown rice.

Almond Flour

A single-ingredient flour, almond flour is often used in baking by the gluten-averse or those wishing for a more densely textured product. It is a good sugar, though barely a sugar at all, with 24 grams of carbohydrates to a cup vs. 86 to a cup of whole wheat flour.

Coconut Flour

Coconut is not a nut but a fruit seed, thus usable by most people with nut allergies. It is a great source of fiber, low in carbohydrates, and high in protein. It is a good sugar.

Rye Flour

Made from whole grain rye kernels, rye flour contains more soluble fiber than wheat flour and thus is slower-acting in the body. It is a good sugar, but be aware that it is often blended with all-purpose flour for commercial sale.

Corn Flour

Milled from dried whole corn grains, this flour contains the hull, the germ, and the endosperm of the corn—contrary to corn starch, which is made from the endosperm only. It is a whole grain flour and therefore a good sugar.

CARBOHYDRATES

The Major Sugar Family

Until now we have been using the word *sugar* in a very broad sense. It is time to get closer to the essence of things. All the sugars we have been discussing, whether they are present in foods with a sweet flavor or contain sugar in the form of starch, belong to the large family of carbohydrates.

Carbohydrates are composed of carbon (C), hydrogen (H), and oxygen (O). These three elements can combine in either simple or complex ways, which will produce different sugars. While chemically speaking they are all sugars, each has its own characteristics that are worth knowing.

THE DIFFERENT KINDS OF CARBOHYDRATES

Carbohydrates can be divided into three major groups, or families, according to the number of molecules that go into their composition: monosaccharides, disaccharides, and polysaccharides. This division into three groups is important as each of these groups contains sugar properties specific to that group.

Monosaccharides

The chemical structure of these sugars is the simplest because they consist of only one single molecule (from the Greek *monos,* meaning "unique").

Glucose and Dextrose

Also known as D-glucose, dextrose is actually crystalline glucose. It is a form of glucose that can be found in abundance in fruits and honey. It is also derived from plants, such as corn, to be used as a sweetener. Glucose is the body's preferred carbohydrate-based energy source. It is the form of sugar found in the bloodstream and required by cells. All other sugars must therefore be transformed into glucose before the body will be able to use them.

Another name for glucose is "grape sugar," because these fruits have a high concentration of it. Grape sugar is mostly of interest to the food and beverage industries and not sold in local markets.

Fructose or Levulose

This form of sugar is also called "fruit sugar," as large amounts of this, too, can be found in fruits. It can also be obtained from the starch of corn and other crops. The fruit sugar sold in stores, therefore, does not always come from fruits, contrary to what the name suggests. In the body, fructose must be turned into glucose by the liver before it can be used for energy, so it's a slower process.

Galactose

This form of sugar is found in milk and other dairy products. Its name is derived from the Greek words for milk and sugar.

? Did You Know?

Because of their extremely simple chemical structure, monosaccharides do not have to be digested in order to be utilizable. They can cross through the intestinal mucous membranes immediately and enter the bloodstream. This is why seriously injured or ill individuals are put on a drip containing a glucose solution.

Generally speaking, monosaccharides are the sugars that are most rapidly available for the muscles.

Based on the speed with which they enter the bloodstream and are available for use by the cell, they have been designated as "fast-acting" sugars. These notions of fast-acting sugar and slow-acting sugar have been called into question today. We will revisit this subject in chapter 11.

In various combinations, the three monosaccharides—glucose, fructose, and galactose—form all the other sugars (the disaccharides and the polysaccharides).

Disaccharides

Disaccharides consist of two monosaccharides.

Maltose or Malt Sugar

This sugar is formed from two glucose molecules. It is especially abundant in malt, which converts from germinated grains, particularly barley.

Lactose or Milk Sugar

This substance breaks down into one glucose molecule and one galactose molecule. One cup of cow's milk contains around

13 grams of lactose. The body uses the intestinal enzyme lactase to break down lactose into glucose and galactose. In cases of lactase deficiency, the body has difficulty with digestion of dairy products.

The medicinal properties of powdered whey for regeneration of the intestinal flora are due in large part to its high lactose content, 50 to 75 percent. (This is not to be confused with whey isolate powder, which contains only 0.1 grams of lactose to 20 grams of powder.)

Sucrose
(Cane Sugar, Beet Sugar)
These additional names are due to the fact that sucrose is present in high quantities in these plants. It is extracted industrially from them to produce the sugar most commonly used today. This sugar is called "whole" if it contains vitamins and minerals, and "refined" if it does not. Sucrose consists of one glucose molecule and one fructose molecule.

Disaccharides are very simple chemical structures and require only extremely minor digestive conversion. Generally speaking, they enter the bloodstream a little more slowly than the direct sugars, or monosaccharides. For this reason they are considered semi-fast-acting sugars.

Polysaccharides
Polysaccharides consist of a very large number of glucose molecules bound together. These molecules form long chains that can contain up to 250,000 units of glucose and are known as "complex" sugars. Grouped together these molecules form starch. There are two different kinds of starches.

Plant Starch

This starch is produced by plants and stored in their cells as an energy reserve. It is especially found in seeds (for example, cereal grains and leguminous plants), tubers (potatoes), root vegetables (celery, cassava), certain fruits (plantains), and tree nuts (such as chestnuts).

Plant starch cannot be used as is by the body. The glucose chains that form plant starch are too long and must first be divided into smaller and smaller segments, then into isolated glucose molecules before they can enter the blood. This division is carried out during the digestive process. It takes place primarily in the mouth, thanks to ptyalin, a digestive sap found in the saliva, and then in the intestine. This process can last as long as several hours. As a general rule, the sugar that is the result of these transformations enters the bloodstream rather slowly. This is why polysaccharides are referred to as slow-acting or delayed sugars.

Animal Starch

Animals and human beings also store fuel reserves in the form of long chains of glucose molecules. The number of these molecules is much lower than those found in plant starch chains; it is around 10,000 units. This animal starch is the glycogen that the body stores in the liver and muscles. Whenever necessary, the body converts the glycogen back into isolated glucose molecules to cover its energy needs.

Cellulose

Cellulose is another polysaccharide. It consists of chains containing 10,000 glucose molecules, but these chains are organized differently from the way they are found in starch. This unique organization is what makes plant fibers rigid. These hard fibers form the plant's support tissue and confer solidity to the husks (bran) of grains, to help protect them from outside attack.

To properly fulfill its role, cellulose must be hard and rigid and not break down easily, for example when it comes into contact with water. Because of its hardness, cellulose cannot be digested by our digestive tract. It remains unconverted and is never absorbed into the body. It forms the substances of ballast and roughage that, by filling the intestinal lumen, encourage intestinal peristalsis.

THE DIFFERENT CARBOHYDRATES

MONOSACCHARIDES (ONE MOLECULE)	DISACCHARIDES (TWO MOLECULES)	POLYSACCHARIDES (NUMEROUS MOLECULES)
Glucose	Maltose (two glucose molecules)	Plant starch (250,000 glucose molecules)
Fructose	Lactose (one glucose + one galactose molecule)	Animal starch (glycogen: 10,000 glucose molecules)
Galactose	Sucrose (one glucose + one fructose molecule)	Cellulose (10,000 glucose molecules)

THE NEED FOR CARBOHYDRATES

Carbohydrates play no role, so to speak, in the construction of the body. They primarily are used to provide the body with the energy it needs to function, regulate the body's temperature, and make physical activity possible.

A variety of experiments have been performed to try to determine what the optimum carbohydrate intake for human beings should be. The figures obtained vary from one study to the next. This is a very difficult question to resolve, as the needs of various individuals can be very different.

In fact, some people possess a basically slow metabolism; they burn little and slowly. Their carbohydrate needs are not so large as those with higher metabolisms. The latter individuals, who could be called restless types, burn through what they eat quite quickly. They need a higher number of carbohydrates.

Another factor is how active an individual's lifestyle is. Some people lead very sedentary lives and thus do not have need for a large amount of fuel. Others perform daily work that requires substantial energy intake. Finally, we should not overlook the role played by stress or its absence. While our needs for sugar are low when all is going well in our lives, they increase quite quickly when we are under pressure and great demands are being made of us.

The daily carbohydrate recommendation has been determined by some researchers to be 40–45 percent of the day's total dietary requirements. Others push this up to 50–55 percent. If expressed in grams, this would represent plus or minus 400 grams a day.

By looking at the carbohydrate content of the primary foods that provide energy, it is easy to see that these needs can be covered quite effortlessly.

AVERAGE CARBOHYDRATE CONTENT OF SEVERAL FOODS

FOOD	CONTENT IN WEIGHT PERCENTAGE
Green vegetables	6
Potatoes	20
Fresh fruits	20
Cooked pasta	30
Cereals (grains)	50
Bread	50
Dried fruits	60
Flour	70
Cookies	70–80
Honey	77

There is actually no real need to calculate our needs for carbohydrates and what that corresponds to in food quantity. Our bodies give us an appetite when extra fuel is needed. During a meal the appetite remains unsatisfied as long as the body indicates a need for more fuel. When it has acquired enough, a sensation of satiety appears, although in some cases we may not initially recognize it. Over the course of the day, when blood sugar goes down the body gives the signal to eat. If the blood sugar level continues to drop, the body urges us to eat food, specifically high-sugar foods.

The blood sugar level is so fundamental in body functioning and well-being that it is helpful to look at how the body is working constantly to maintain blood sugar at its optimum level.

BLOOD SUGAR LEVEL

Variations and Regulation

The body needs a steady supply of fuel, which can fluctuate depending on the demands of individual functions.

GLYCEMIA

The billions of cells that make up our bodies are dependent on glucose to carry out their roles in the body. Consequently, the bloodstream must always carry a sufficient quantity of glucose so that the cells will be able to draw from it at any time according to their needs. The body provides for this need by maintaining a constant rate of glucose in the blood.

The content of glucose in the blood is the blood sugar level or, more clinically, glycemia. It is around 1 gram per liter of blood. This rate tends to be steady with predictable variations. For example, blood sugar levels are lower when someone is hungry and rise after a meal. Once freed by digestion, the many carbohydrates that were consumed cross through the walls of the intestines and make their way into the bloodstream. This inevitably ensures a rise in the level of blood sugar.

Blood sugar levels can also drop, for example during intense and sudden physical exertion. The great demand placed on the muscles by this effort increases their need for glucose. Stress has the same effect: it increases the rate of combustion and lowers sugar content in the blood.

On an empty stomach, blood sugar levels are considered normal if they are between 72 mg/dl and 108 mg/dl. The blood sugar level after a meal is still considered normal if two hours later it is between 100 mg/dl and 140 mg/dl.

☞ Good to Know

When blood sugar levels are good, we feel good, full of vim and vigor. We are able to think clearly and are in a good mood. We are not hungry and do not crave sweets.

A blood sugar level that is too high is *hyper*glycemia; a level that is too low is *hypo*glycemia. Readings below 72 mg/dl and above 108 mg/dl are not within normal parameters, and the individual is not physiologically healthy. An abnormal blood sugar level (too low or too high) does not have any truly onerous consequences so long as it is only temporary, such as before or after a meal. But if it is of any duration, physiological disorders will inevitably arise in all cases. In fact, the body is no more capable of tolerating excess sugar than it is of tolerating sugar deficiency.

Hyperglycemia

Hyperglycemia starts when the blood sugar level goes above 108 mg/dl. The increase can be small 1.8 g/l, middling (2.5 g/l), or quite high (5 to 6 g/l). Abnormally high quantities of sugar in the blood will alter blood composition substantially. Among the first symptoms of hyperglycemia are great fatigue and feelings of drowsiness. Because sugar is fuel for the body, this loss of energy may seem surprising. The fact is, any change in blood composition will reduce the body's functional capacities and rob it of energy.

> Excess sugar is an assault and forces the body to fight. It mobilizes all its strength for this battle and becomes exhausted.

If the blood has too high a glucose content, the body will begin looking for ways to get rid of it. It will eliminate as much as possible through the kidneys in the urine. Frequent urination and the presence of sugar in urine are therefore symptoms of hyperglycemia.

📖 A Little History

In antiquity, physicians tasted the urine of their patients to make a diagnosis. If it had a sweet flavor, they would deduce that the patient was suffering from hyperglycemia and diabetes. Other physicians asked patients to urinate near an anthill. If the ants quickly fell upon a patient's urine, it was likely high in sugar.

The body also tries to reduce the intensity of the assault on its tissues that excess sugar represents by diluting it to the maximum extent possible. It triggers intense feelings of thirst that prompt the individual suffering from hyperglycemia to drink large quantities of fluids. The abundant amount of liquid ingested dilutes the blood and cellular fluids. It also encourages the elimination of glucose by the urine, by supplying an increased medium for transporting it out of the body.

Other disorders associated with hyperglycemia include problems with eyesight, headaches, itchy skin, dry tongue, nausea, and brain fog.

SYMPTOMS OF HYPERGLYCEMIA

- Great fatigue, drowsiness
- Need to urinate more frequently
- Sugar in the urine
- Increase in the quantity of urine eliminated
- Thirst, sensation of dry mouth
- Fuzzy vision
- Headaches
- Itchy skin
- Nausea
- Brain fog

Hypoglycemia

The lower boundary of normal blood sugar levels is around 72 mg/dl.

When the blood sugar level drops below this benchmark figure, the body begins to experience a loss of fuel, which is known as hypoglycemia. A sense of weariness settles in and an urgent need to eat makes itself felt. This prompts the person to eat in order to restore a healthy blood sugar level.

If no carbohydrate intake occurs and energy expenditures continue, the blood sugar level will continue to fall. At 0.65 g/l, feelings of fatigue become pronounced and the desire to eat moves its target from food in general to sweet foods in particular. This transition is precise and acute. If no sugar is provided to the body and the blood sugar level falls to 0.6 g/l or lower, it is no longer a simple case of hypoglycemia but a full-blown hypoglycemic crisis.

Because of the deficit of fuel the person now feels extremely fatigued, even exhausted. In such a crisis the person no longer has any strength and feels too weak to make any kind of effort. Everything seems so overwhelming that an individual in this state can even begin to panic, because life truly seems too difficult. Because the brain needs glucose to function properly, the individual becomes nervous, anxious, agitated, impatient, and confused. Concentrating and speaking becomes difficult, and the cardiac muscle struggles to perform its work. The legs start to feel like jelly, and there may be palpitations and dizzy spells that can lead to losing consciousness. All of these symptoms are still accompanied by an irresistible hunger for something sweet. The signal is clear that carbohydrate intake is imperative and urgent.

SYMPTOMS OF HYPOGLYCEMIA

- Great fatigue, lack of energy, sensation of extreme weakness
- Strong craving for sweet foods
- Nervousness, anxiety, agitation
- Mental confusion, impossible to concentrate, difficulty speaking
- Headache, nausea, blurred vision
- Palpitations, perspiration, pallor, trembling, vertigo, loss of consciousness

VARIATIONS IN BLOOD SUGAR LEVEL

g/liter of glucose

5	Very strong hyperglycemia
	Semi-strong hyperglycemia
2.5	Hyperglycemia
1.4	Normal blood sugar level
1.1	Normal level on an empty stomach
0.8	Hypoglycemia
0.6	Crisis of hypoglycemia

The body works constantly to maintain a normal blood sugar level, and as we'll see, it is quick to react when this level rises into hyperglycemic levels or falls into hypoglycemia.

REGULATION OF HYPERGLYCEMIA

As our food is digested, the glucose it contains is released into the intestines and passes through the intestinal walls to enter the bloodstream. This causes the blood sugar level to rise gradually. When it reaches the upper limit of normal blood sugar and threatens to go beyond it, the pancreas goes into a state of alert. It is the organ most responsible for fighting against hyperglycemia. Moreover, it is the only organ in the body that can take this kind of responsive action, although there are several glands that can come into play to correct cases of hypoglycemia.

The pancreas is located on the left side of the abdomen at the same level as the liver, which it faces. Since it releases digestive juices into the intestines, it is considered to be a digestive gland. But the pancreas also has an endocrine function (hormonal), as do the thyroid and pituitary glands. It is this function that concerns us here, because the pancreas produces the hormone insulin.

The quantities of insulin produced by the pancreas are always adapted to what the body needs, so there is a small amount for a slightly boosted blood sugar level, but much more when the normal limit has been vastly surpassed. The effect of the insulin that enters the bloodstream is to make the cells in the muscles and liver absorb the glucose in the blood and convert it into glycogen to be stored as an energy reserve. In short, glucose is the form in which the energy is transported and utilized, and glycogen is the form in which it is stored. The quantity of glucose that can be set aside as a reserve in this way can go up to 300 or 400 grams.

When the glycogen reserves are full, they can no longer store any additional glucose. The insulin that was released to correct the hyperglycemia will then no longer transform the glucose into glycogen but into fat that will be stored in the adipocytes, connective tissue cells that are specialized for the storing of energy reserves in the form of lipids. This kind of storing is physiologically appropriate because a certain amount of fat is necessary for the body to function well. However, in cases where overeating is an issue, this stored fat can become excessive and lead to harmful weight gain.

The action of insulin therefore transforms excess sugar into glycogens and then fat. While the first of these stored energy reserves is quickly and easily converted back into glucose when it is needed, the same is not true for fat. Its conversion is slower and more difficult.

THE CONVERSION OF GLUCOSE IN HYPERGLYCEMIA

ENDOCRINE GLAND	HORMONE	RESERVE TYPE
Pancreas	Insulin	Glycogen in the liver and muscles
Pancreas	Insulin	Fat in the adipocytes

REGULATION OF HYPOGLYCEMIA

Our daily activities are constantly burning away the glucose present in the bloodstream, making it inevitable that its level will drop. When the blood sugar level falls below the minimal rate (0.8 g/l) and reaches the crisis stage of hypoglycemia (0.6 g/l and lower), corrective phenomena are called into action. If they do not intervene, a hypoglycemic crisis will occur. This state is characterized by great physical and mental fatigue, one that does not permit the individual to perform normal activity.

The body has several different options for correcting hypoglycemic imbalance but only one for hyperglycemia, because it is more urgent to correct an energy deficit than a surplus. If nothing is done the body will quickly find itself in difficulty, if not in actual danger. The individual can no longer deal with the situation and has no defenses. This is less so in the case of hyperglycemia, where an individual can continue to act, meet obligations, and maintain defenses. It is therefore a much less urgent situation, but the long-term harmful effects of hyperglycemia can also be quite serious.

As we have seen, the first way the body has to correct hypoglycemia is to prompt the person to eat food in order to increase the blood sugar level. Hunger pangs appear when the blood sugar level falls below 0.8 g/l. This is initially a hunger for any kind of food, but the further the blood sugar level falls, the greater this craving changes into a specific and insistent desire for sugar. In fact, if the lack of sugar is minimal, the digestion of any kind of food will rapidly provide the body with the glucose it needs. Conversely, when the lack of sugar is more pronounced and the situation has become more urgent, the body requires sweet foods. The fast-acting sugars this food contains will swiftly find their way into the bloodstream and restore the proper blood sugar level.

While eating is the most logical and natural means of correcting hypoglycemia, there is one drawback: food is not always available. In a situation in which the body does not have the benefit of an ingested sugar, it needs to seek elsewhere. The sole remaining option at its disposal is to find it within, from the glycogen and fats that have been stored in its tissues. The conversion of these energy reserves into glucose is made possible thanks to the action of various endocrine glands.

One of these glands is the pancreas. When hypoglycemia occurs, it releases the hormone glucagon. This hormone works on the glycogen stored in the liver and muscles and transforms it into glucose.

Two other endocrine glands function in the same way. The adrenal glands release adrenaline, which accelerates all the body's organic processes to enable it to better defend itself when threatened. The thyroid gland releases thyroxine, a hormone that stimulates the consumption of oxygen and the basic metabolism of all the cells and tissues in the body.

Thanks to these three glands, glucose is extracted from the glycogen reserves. But these reserves are not always full, and consequently, depending on the circumstances, they can be depleted. If there is not enough glucose from this source, the body will have to turn to another kind of energy reserve: fats that have been stored in the adipocytes. The conversion of fat into glucose is made thanks to the hormone somatotropin, which is released by the anterior pituitary gland. This substance enters the bloodstream and causes the glucose level to climb.

THE CONVERSION OF GLYCOGEN AND FAT INTO GLUCOSE IN CASES OF HYPOGLYCEMIA

ENDOCRINE GLAND	HORMONE	RESERVE TYPE CONVERTED
Pancreas	Glucagon	Glycogen of the liver and muscles
Adrenals	Adrenaline	Glycogen of the liver and muscles
Thyroid	Thyroxine	Glycogen of the liver and muscles
Pituitary gland	Somatotropin	Fats in the adipocytes
Adrenals	Glucocorticoids	Proteins

In an attempt to counter hypoglycemia the body still has one final defense system it can turn to when the aforementioned methods are insufficient: glucose can be found, to a small extent, in protein composition. In extreme cases the body can gain access to these glucose molecules by breaking up muscle protein. The glucose that has been freed in this way will be fed into the bloodstream, where it will raise the blood sugar level. The hormones used to break down proteins are the glucocorticoids, a class of steroid hormones secreted by the adrenal glands.

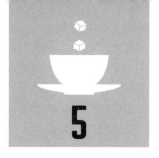

5

DISEASES CAUSED BY BAD SUGARS

From Deficiencies to Diabetes

The regular and generous consumption of refined sugar and flour is the root cause of numerous illnesses afflicting the "modern human." As the human body was not designed for their ingestion by nature, these fake foods attack our organism and disrupt its functioning. Here are the principal diseases that result from the consumption of bad sugars.

STARVATION OF THE BODY

To function normally, and consequently enjoy good health, the body uses around fifty nutrients, primarily vitamins, minerals, trace elements, and amino acids. These nutrients are absolutely essential to the body and must be supplied by the food that is consumed. This is due to the fact that the body is incapable of producing them by itself.

It so happens that while these foods offered to us by nature can supply all the nutrients we need, this is no longer the case when these foods have been adulterated. Because they have been stripped of a portion of their component parts, these foods are now deficient. When they are consumed, the nutrients they no longer contain will now also be missing from the body, and a deficiency will occur.

The deficiencies in foods that are essential for the construction and repair of tissues can lead to weakening of and damage to the organs. When there is a deficit in the nutrients that are necessary for the functioning of the body, the organs can no longer perform their tasks as well as they should. Their functioning can either slow down, be performed incompletely or poorly, or even come to a complete halt.

The refining of sugar and grains removes a large number of nutrients from these foods. The table found on page 24 shows the difference between whole sugar (with blackstrap molasses), raw sugar (without blackstrap molasses but still containing some nutrients), and refined white table sugar, the latter of which is devoid of nutritional value. Contrary to whole sugar, refined white sugar contains no proteins or vitamins, and its mineral content is close to zero.

The differences in the composition of refined flour and whole grain flour are also extremely important.

VITAMIN CONTENT OF DIFFERENT FLOURS (IN MG)

	VITAMIN B$_1$	VITAMIN B$_2$	NIACIN	VITAMIN B$_6$
Whole Grain Flour	0.36	0.24	5	0.40
Refined All-Purpose Flour	0.10	0.08	0.6	0.20

MINERAL CONTENT OF
DIFFERENT GRAINS (IN MG)

	POTASSIUM	SODIUM	CALCIUM	MAGNESIUM	IRON	TOTAL
Whole Wheat Flour	400	40	40	120	15	615
All-Purpose White Flour	12	8	15	17	1.3	53.3
Whole Rice	560	160	10	250	50	1130
White Rice (bran removed)	62	14	8	23	3	110

In all-purpose white flour there are two times less vitamin B_6; three times less vitamins B_1, B_2, and calcium; six times less magnesium; twelve times less iron, and thirty-three times less potassium than in whole grain flour. Some refined flours may have a higher vitamin content, but these are synthetic vitamins that have been added to "fortify" the flour, and their nutritive value is less than that of vitamins from food.

The problem is identical when it comes to cereal grains. Similar differences of composition can be found between white rice and brown rice. In fact, an individual who is consuming only products made from all-purpose flour or other refined grains is deprived of 70 percent of the most valuable substances that grains contain. So instead of regularly receiving the required nutrients, people who regularly eat white bread, refined sugar, pasta made from all-purpose refined flour, white rice, and so on are actually depriving themselves of these valuable substances.

The net result of these combined deficiencies inevitably is an escalating number of increasingly intense disruptions of regular body functions. Over time they will lead to organic lesions.

☞ Good to Know

Diseases caused by deficiencies are related to the nutrients the body is lacking. A deficiency of magnesium, for example, will produce a weakening of the nervous system, leg cramps, a drop in the body's resistance to infections, and formation of cancerous tumors over time. Deficiencies of the B vitamins will reduce the body's energy production, resistance to stress, regeneration of the blood, and so forth.

The risk of deficiencies is reinforced by the fact that deficient foods not only no longer provide the body with nutrients but they strip nutrients already present in the body. The expression "vitamin thieves" is used to describe this situation. Normally each item of food supplies the vitamins that are required by the enzymes responsible for transforming them to a form usable by the body. When food is deficient in these vitamins, this is no longer the case. So that biochemical transformations can continue to take place despite this lack, the body has to provide the missing vitamins to the enzymes. The body ends up being even more deficient, with these deficiencies added to those created externally. If certain enzymes are also deficient, that adds still another layer of difficulty.

ACIDIFICATION OF THE TERRAIN

If we are to enjoy good heath, a balance must exist between the acid and alkaline substances in our bodies. This is known as the acid-alkaline balance, and when it is functioning properly, the enzymes responsible for all biochemical transformations can perform their tasks perfectly well. This in turn allows each cell and organ to perform its own work properly, thereby assuring the health and vitality of the body.

The consumption of refined sugar and flour disrupts the acid-alkaline balance of the body by increasing the production of acids. The resulting acidification of the body's cellular terrain prevents the enzymes from performing their work properly, which in turn leads to the manifestation of many health problems.

The Mechanisms of Acid Production

Refined sugars and flours provide glucose to the body. Once in the body, for example in the muscles, this glucose must undergo a series of transformations to provide energy.

During the *anaerobic phase* (without oxygen), glucose is attacked by enzymes and transformed into citric acid, which is then attacked by other enzymes that transform it into alpha-ketoglutaric acid (or a-ketoglutaric acid). This in turn is transformed into other acids, called intermediary toxic metabolites (ITM). Although toxic to the body, their presence is only temporary.

In the *aerobic phase* that follows, which is in the presence of oxygen and under the effect of other enzymes, the final acid of the series, lactic acid, is transformed into energy and ceases to exist in the acid state. The sole residues that remain are carbon dioxide and water.

TRANSFORMATION OF GLUCOSE INTO ENERGY

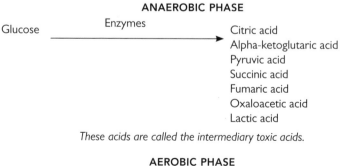

ANAEROBIC PHASE

Glucose ——— Enzymes ———→ Citric acid
Alpha-ketoglutaric acid
Pyruvic acid
Succinic acid
Fumaric acid
Oxaloacetic acid
Lactic acid

These acids are called the intermediary toxic acids.

AEROBIC PHASE

ITM + Oxygen ——— Enzymes ———→ $H_2O + CO_2$ + energy

Glucose is, strictly speaking, a clean energy. It is not supposed to produce waste products that collect in the body and make it sick. However, the bulk of the sugar and flour we consume is refined and lacks the vitamins and trace elements necessary for activating essential enzymes. The transformation of glucose into energy is not carried to its intended conclusion but interrupted during one of the intermediary toxic metabolic stages. Consequently, instead of benefiting from the energy (glucose) it requires to function properly, the body is given toxins in the form of citric acid, alpha-ketoglutaric acid, or any of the other intermediary toxic acids, depending just when the series of transformations is interrupted. There is no production of energy, but there is production of acids. These acids collect and lay the groundwork for future diseases.

The Three Harmful Effects of Acids

Acids attack the tissues, injuring and inflaming them, which can lead to rheumatism, tendinitis, neuritis, eczema, and other maladies.

Acids demineralize the tissues, forcing other parts of the body to surrender large quantities of minerals to neutralize the surplus acids. This can result in the decalcification of the skeletal structure, arthritis, tooth decay, dry eczema, lower blood pressure and energy levels, greater tendency to feel fatigued and/or depressed, and so on.

Acids reduce the body's defenses, leaving the immune system unable to fight as efficiently against infections such as flu, colds, and cystitis, and against allergies such as hay fever.

THE POISONING OF THE BODY

Normal body function produces metabolic residues and wastes that are known as toxins. Normally these toxins are eliminated at the same rate they are produced via the five emunctory organs of elimination: liver, intestines, kidneys, skin, and lungs. When these organs can no longer manage to properly expel toxins from the body, they start accumulating in the body, or more specifically, in the body's cellular terrain.

From the natural medicine perspective, this accumulation of toxins constitutes the principal cause of disease. The presence of these wastes in the blood, cells, and organs prevents them from functioning normally, which creates increasingly severe health problems the more the amount of toxins in the organism rises.

The presence of toxins thickens the blood and prevents it from flowing properly. The toxins are then deposited on the walls of the vessels and to some extent in the organs through which the blood flows (the liver, the brain). They cause congestion that disrupts the ability of the organs to function properly. While some toxins cause problems for the body simply because of their presence, others do so because of their aggressive nature. Many toxins irritate the body tissues and trigger inflammation, followed by sclerosis, which is abnormal hardening of the tissue. They can also alter the genetic material of the cells, which is one way cancer can develop.

There are two major kinds of toxins, crystal and colloidal. Crystals are toxins whose angular form and hard consistency causes inflammation and lesions. The acids we discussed above belong to this category of toxins. They are caused by proteins as well as by refined sugar. The illnesses they cause have been described above.

Colloidal toxins are soft, shapeless substances, such as cholesterol and mucus, that congest the organs and obstruct the passageways. They are formed from the starch of grains in general (bread, pasta, rice, and so on), most especially when these grains have been refined. Polyunsaturated fats and trans fats are another potential source of colloidal toxins.

DISEASES CAUSED BY COLLOIDAL TOXINS

Ingesting too much food made from refined grains can make the body ill due to the extreme quantity of colloidal substances that will then take up residence in the body's cellular terrain.

Cardiovascular Diseases

The thickening of the blood by colloidal toxins leads to poor circulation (heavy legs, cramps), formation of deposits in the blood vessels (arteriosclerosis), distention of the walls of blood vessels (varicose veins, hemorrhoids), and obstruction of the vessels (heart attacks, strokes).

The reason many people take prescription blood thinners is simply that their blood is too thick.

Hepatic (Liver) Weakness

The liver is the primary organ responsible for neutralizing colloidal toxins and eliminating them once they have been diluted by bile. If the quantity of colloidal substances is too high, the liver becomes exhausted and no longer secretes sufficient bile. This eventually leads to digestive problems, constipation, and so forth. Another consequence of a weakened liver is a reduction of its ability to store glucose in the form of glycogen so that it can convert it back into glucose when needed.

Respiratory Ailments

When the liver does not manage to eliminate colloidal toxins, the respiratory tract picks up the slack. It serves as a kind of safety conduit for eliminating any overflow. However, the respiratory passages can also be deluged by these wastes and become congested. The result of this situation will be colds, sinusitis, bronchitis, or asthma.

Skin Disorders

Another emunctory organ for colloidal waste is the skin, or to be more specific, the sebaceous glands. When the glands are congested by too large a quantity of colloidal waste, whitehead pimples, oozing eczema, acne, boils, sties, and even sebaceous cysts may appear.

OBESITY—STORED SUGAR AS FAT

Every time a person eats sugar and the blood sugar level rises, the pancreas releases insulin to bring that level back to normal. The excess sugar is transformed into glycogen that is stored in the liver and the muscles. When these reserves are full, the sugar is no longer transformed into glycogen but into fat, which is stockpiled in specialized cells: the adipocytes.

The adipocytes are spread throughout all the tissues of the body, but some have a larger reserve than others. They resemble pockets with extendable walls that allow them to increase their size in order to store more fat.

It is the increase in the volume of the adipocytes that leads to the dilation of tissues that are a typical feature of overweight people. The weight gain is minor in the beginning and increases with the passage of time (and the consumption of sugar). When the body's weight goes beyond what is considered normal body weight for one's size by 25 percent, it is considered obese.

The transformation of sugar into fat and the resulting

weight gain is dependent on secretions of insulin. The release of insulin is greater and faster if the carbohydrates consumed are fast-acting sugars. This explains how obesity is directly related to bad sugars.

> The current "epidemic" of obesity is predominant in the populations that consume bad sugars and fats, rather than among those whose diet is closer to nature and includes good sugars.

Unfortunately the role played by bad sugars does not stop there. The releases of insulin that are triggered by their consumption encourage not only the storage of fat created by sugar but the storage of all fats, meaning all those present in the foods that are eaten at the same time a person is ingesting a bad sugar; for example, the fat present in milk chocolate or pastry cream. Therefore, putting on weight is primarily the result of eating bad sugars.

☝ Good to Know

Dietary fats that are absorbed during meals are stored in their own distinctive rhythm. This rhythm is intensified by the presence of insulin, so when the body is permeated with insulin, many more dietary fats are stored. This is almost always the case for those who habitually consume bad sugars.

Deposits of Cellulitis

When colloidal wastes and fats overfill the adipocytes under the skin, the latter increase in size and become apparent.

DIABETES—
PERSISTENT HYPERGLYCEMIA

The consumption of foods high in carbohydrates inevitably creates a temporary state of hyperglycemia. When the glucose that has triggered this rise in blood sugar level comes from foods with good sugars, it enters the bloodstream slowly and the blood sugar level does not rise too high or too quickly. The reaction of the pancreas is gentle and the quantity of insulin it releases is exactly what is required.

When bad sugars are the cause of hyperglycemia, the pancreas reacts violently. In fact, bad sugar enters the bloodstream in large quantities and causes the blood sugar level to rapidly rise quite high. The pancreas then swiftly releases a large amount of insulin in response. Because hyperglycemia is experienced as a fierce attack and a threat to the balance of the body, sometimes more insulin than necessary is released.

This exaggerated reaction does not have any adverse consequences if it only happens once in a while. However, when it takes place repeatedly over the course of the day and occurs day after day, it tires the pancreas and eventually exhausts it. This is very often the case in contemporary culture. Many people consume primarily bad sugars in great quantities and repeatedly over the day, every day. The exhausted pancreas can no longer manage the amount of insulin that's needed, or what it does produce is inferior in quality. The excess sugar that is present in the bloodstream during hyperglycemia cannot then be evacuated. It does not make its way into the cells but remains in the bloodstream and collects there. This is diabetes.

The various symptoms of diabetes are manifestations of the body's efforts to eliminate surplus sugar or of its suffering from being poisoned by this sugar.

Symptoms of Diabetes

Elimination of Sugar in Urine (Glycosuria)

Normally urine contains no glucose, but when blood sugar levels are consistently too high, the body protects itself by eliminating some of this excess sugar via the urine.

Increase in the Quantity of Urine Expelled (Polyuria)

The high concentration of urine—due to the presence of glucose—triggers an osmotic mechanism that draws water into the urinary system in order to dilute the urine. The result is that diabetics eliminate larger quantities of urine.

Intense and Excessive Thirst (Polydipsia)

The fluid that has been drawn from the tissues to dilute the urine causes a shortage of fluid in the cells. The body experiences the sensation of thirst, which stimulates a desire to drink in order to compensate for the deficiency of liquid.

Intense Appetite (Polyphagia)

The intense craving for food is caused by the permanent lack of glucose on the cellular level (the sugar is remaining in the bloodstream), combined with the abundant diuresis (production of urine) that is responsible for the high loss of minerals that need to be replaced.

Acidosis or Ketoacidosis

When the autolysis process, which takes place on the cellular level, is substantial, the breakdown of fatty substances into glucose does not continue to take place properly because this breakdown requires the presence of glucose to be effective. The transformation of the fatty substances stops at the acid stage (acetone, ketonic acids). When they collect in the bloodstream, the ketonic substances make the blood acidic (acidosis). Alkaline minerals can neutralize them, but when there is too great a quantity of acids, the body is not able to provide enough of them. The blood then quickly becomes increasingly acidic (acetone crisis). This state is very dangerous because it is the equivalent of poisoning the body with acetone, a toxin that plunges the individual into a deep and dangerous sleep—the diabetic coma.

Only the consumption of sweet foods at the onset of the crisis or an injection of glucose can stop this crisis and save the patient.

Sclerosis of the Blood Vessels

Sclerosis (or hardening) of the vessels is due to the aggressive nature of the sugar concentrations present in the bloodstream. This occurs particularly at the extremities (open sores, gangrene), the eyes, and the kidneys.

Prone to Infection

A terrain that is oversaturated with wastes (or with unnecessary sugar) is favorable for germs. The general lack of resistance against the assault of germs manifests in local infections (boils, sties) or generalized ones.

Nerve Disorders

The attack on the nerves by acids produced by sugar triggers polyneuritis and nervous lesions.

Skin Disorders
These can be infections, boils, and so forth.

Hyperglycemic Crisis
The major danger that threatens diabetics is the sudden hyperglycemic crisis. After ingesting too many carbohydrates, for example, in a situation where the secretions of insulin are insufficient, the rate of sugar in the blood can increase catastrophically. The imbalance of the blood composition can become so extreme that the body is no longer able to function normally. The patient falls into a coma (diabetic coma) and will die if no treatment is applied (injection of insulin and hypoglycemic agents) to bring down the level of sugar.

Types of Diabetes
There are two types of diabetes, and both are related to overconsumption of bad sugars. There may also be a genetic predisposition.

Type 1 Diabetes
This type of diabetes is characterized by an insufficiency in the quantity of insulin produced by the pancreas, which is required for cells to absorb glucose from the bloodstream. Because the sugar is unable to make its way into the cells, the body autolyzes (digests or breaks down) its own tissues to produce some, which causes the patient to lose weight. This is sometimes referred to as "thin diabetes," and in the days before insulin therapy, it was eventually and inevitably fatal.

Type 2 Diabetes
In this kind of diabetes the quantity of insulin released is sufficient in relation to the body's needs, but it fails to properly per-

form its function. Sugar stagnates in the body and is not used. This form of the disease is characterized by inordinate weight gain, hence its nickname "fat diabetes."

Both forms of diabetes have as a primary cause the excessive consumption of bad sugar. Proof of this can be found in the fact that diabetes is unknown to people living a traditional lifestyle close to nature and who therefore do not consume refined sugar or grains but only whole grains and other foods containing good sugars.

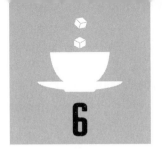

6

REACTIVE HYPOGLYCEMIA

Body Disturbances and
Sugar Dependency

Standard incidences of hypoglycemia occur when the intake of carbohydrates is not substantial enough to compensate for losses due to physical exertion or stress. There is another kind of glycemia, however: reactive glycemia. It is caused by a disproportionate reaction of the pancreas when dealing with the arrival of bad sugars. To understand how this is possible, we must now discuss insulin in greater detail.

Normally the quantity of insulin sent into the bloodstream by the pancreas corresponds precisely to what is necessary to bring the blood sugar level back to normal. This is how blood sugar levels above 1.4 g/l are gradually brought down to around 1 g/l. In this way, we move from a state of hyperglycemia to a normal blood sugar level (curve 1 on the chart on page 74). Sometimes, however—because of the consumption of bad sugars—the quantity of insulin released is more than what is required. This greater amount then has a greater effect, and it is excessive. It causes the rate of blood sugar to fall not just to normal levels, but to plummet even lower (see curve 2 on the same chart). For example, the blood sugar level first drops from 4 g/l to 1 g/l, which is normal, but because of the excess insulin, it continues to fall. It reaches 0.8 g/l, the bottom limit of normal blood sugar level, but instead of stabilizing it keeps falling and reaches 0.5 g/l or less, which is equivalent to a crisis state of pronounced hypoglycemia.

A person who is experiencing hyperglycemia due to the consumption of bad sugars can therefore arrive in a very short time in a state of hypoglycemia, because of the excessive release of insulin. After having too much sugar in the blood, now the individual no longer has enough! A craving for sweets then naturally appears to inspire this person to eat. This kind of hypoglycemia is due to a reaction of the pancreas, which is why it's called reactive hypoglycemia.

But here is where it can get tricky. If the person decides to restore energy by eating more bad sugars, the blood sugar level will climb. The empty and tired feelings will disappear, but this will only last a short while. Very soon the person will be in hypoglycemia again. If bad sugars are resorted to again, the pancreas will again react forcefully and the infernal cycle will be triggered anew. This is why phases of hyperglycemia and hypoglycemia alternate abnormally all day for some people.

The curve of their blood sugar level resembles the Rocky Mountains. They climb steeply toward high peaks, then plunge into the depths, only to climb again toward another peak. And on and on it continues.

While a normal blood sugar curve is fairly horizontal and stable, the curve for people who consume bad sugars resembles the peaks and valleys of a mountain range.

REACTIVE HYPOGLYCEMIA

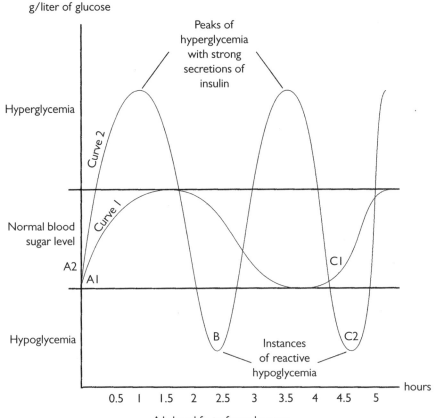

g/liter of glucose

Peaks of hyperglycemia with strong secretions of insulin

Hyperglycemia

Curve 2

Curve 1

Normal blood sugar level

A2

A1

Hypoglycemia

B

C1

C2

Instances of reactive hypoglycemia

hours

0.5   1   1.5   2   2.5   3   3.5   4   4.5   5

A1: breakfast of good sugars
A2: breakfast of bad sugars
B: snack of bad sugars
C1: lunch of good sugars
C2: lunch of bad sugars

The examination of these curves shows that someone experiencing reactive hypoglycemia will be in a hypoglycemic crisis several times a day. Everything will take place differently if instead of bad sugars good ones are eaten, such as those supplied by an apple, for example. The blood sugar level will climb slowly and the pancreas will not have to react forcefully. There will be no hypoglycemia and no craving for sweets.

A HYPERACTIVE PANCREAS

The excessive secretion of insulin is due to the speed and quantity of the sugar entering the bloodstream when food containing bad sugars is consumed. Over the long term, this type of consumption will eventually cause the pancreas to malfunction. This disruption of its functioning is more likely if the body's demands for insulin are always urgent.

When the sugar consumed is a bad sugar that causes the blood sugar level to quickly soar, the pancreas becomes accustomed to releasing insulin very quickly and forcefully. Over time this organ will develop an extreme sensitivity to the presence of bad sugars. When this happens, no sooner will the bad sugars enter the body then the pancreas will go on a state of alert. Instead of releasing insulin gently and in a quantity that meets the needs of the body, it will release a large quantity with great speed. This hyperreactivity will eventually become second nature. But by releasing more insulin than necessary, it causes a steep drop in the blood sugar level and places the individual into a state of pronounced reactive hypoglycemia.

Some people acquire this hypersensitivity and hyperreactivity over the course of their lives because they overindulge in foods containing bad sugars. However, this weakness can also be passed down genetically and manifest from infancy. In both cases the pancreas is more prompt to react and it also takes the same approach to small quantities of bad sugars. Such people are therefore very easily and too often subject to attacks of reactive hypoglycemia.

An additional reason for the dysfunction of the pancreas is that the other organs responsible for maintaining normal blood sugar level are no longer doing their job or are performing it poorly. The pancreas must then take on a greater share of the workload, which leads it to exaggerate its reactions. Among these organs we must include the liver. Overworked by a diet that is too heavy in carbohydrates (but also in fats and proteins), it is no longer capable of transforming glucose into glycogen. Too much glucose remains in the bloodstream and the pancreas must step in to reduce the rate.

The adrenal glands can also contribute to making the pancreas hyperreactive. Overindulgence in coffee, black tea, chocolate, and tobacco stimulates the production of adrenaline, the effect of which is to increase the liver's conversion of glycogen back into glucose. This latter substance, because of the strength of the request, will enter the bloodstream in a large quantity. The blood sugar quickly soars as a result and this obliges the pancreas to take equally strong measures.

Reactive hypoglycemia creates disturbances on the physical and mental levels that are more serious and troubling than those due to normal hypoglycemia. The descriptions of the symptoms of reactive hypoglycemia will appear exaggerated and caricatured to many people, but they are not. Those who suffer from this condition can confirm this. The disturbances caused by reactive hypoglycemia manifest as appetite problems, physical ailments, and mental disorders.

🖐 Good to Know

The hyperreactivity of the pancreas is not acquired in a single day; it is a process that takes place over a period of time, and all who suffer from reactive hypoglycemia are not afflicted to the same degree. During the first stages of the disorder, only weak symptoms appear and only now and then, whereas at an advanced stage, the symptoms appear intensely and often.

THE EXCESSIVE DESIRE FOR SUGAR

In cases of reactive hypoglycemia, the lack of sugar is considerable, and consequently the desire to eat sweets is pronounced. Depending on the intensity of the reactivity of the pancreas, this craving can be strong, extreme, all-consuming, or uncontrollable.

The person undergoing an attack of reactive hypoglycemia feels an imperative need to eat immediately, without waiting another second. The need is so urgent that people in this condition search feverishly for something sweet to ingest. When the disturbance of the pancreas is minor, the person can eat whatever is found, more or less calmly. But if the pancreas is extremely reactive—meaning that there is a huge lack of sugar—the individual will pounce on anything edible. For example, instead of a package of cookies being calmly opened, it gets ripped open as if it were a matter of life or death. The individual will not calmly eat the cookies one by one, but will devour several at a time at top speed, as if trying to eat the largest possible amount of food as quickly as possible.

🖐 Good to Know

The feeling of urgency experienced during a reactive hypoglycemia attack will cause people to forget all they ever knew about good manners. If an attack comes on before a meal, they will sit down at the table and begin eating without waiting for the other guests. Their greed prevents them from exerting any self-control and waiting; it compels them to start filling themselves right away.

The hunger felt by people who have been deeply afflicted by this condition is not only excessive; it is also insatiable. They cannot stop eating continually, all day long. They will not eat for short spells of time, but those times are only the better to prepare them to devour something else. They never seem sated. They can eat more than enough and yet it never seems to satisfy them for long. They quickly begin feeling hungry again and start eating something or other. Their ability to eat astounds all those around them. They give other people the impression that they are constantly eating. In reality, there are times of the day when they do not eat. These occur during the short periods of hyperglycemia during which their need for sugar is satisfied and they are not craving sweets. But these periods are quite brief, lasting from thirty to sixty minutes rather than several hours. All the rest of the time they are in a hypoglycemic state. This gives them an irresistible desire to eat, so they eat.

The disorders described here are due to bad sugars. Things do not play out this way when good sugars are being eaten. Their consumption does not create the desire to continuously eat more sweets. To the contrary, they reduce the craving for sugar. As soon as the body receives the fuel it was missing, a feeling of satiety is established. For example, someone feeling tired decides to eat apples. As the first apple is being eaten, the need for sugar diminishes. By the second or third apple, the need and craving have vanished completely. Nothing is pushing this individual to continue eating—or, more precisely, overeating—as would be the case if foods with bad sugars had been chosen instead.

It is only the bad sugars that, due to their strong effect on the pancreas, short-circuit the feeling of being sated and simply create the desire to eat more sugar. This unhappy chain of circumstances has been summed up in the saying "Bad sugars summon more bad sugars." This is basic knowledge that everyone should have. Someone who eats a chocolate bar or a piece of candy will always be tempted to eat a second piece, then a third, and so on. To get free of the bad sugar cycle it is therefore necessary to abstain and replace them with good sugars.

The strong cravings for sugar felt by people experiencing reactive hypoglycemia should not be taken as signs of self-indulgence or gluttony. Gourmands eat for pleasure; their hunger is aroused by thoughts or the sight of food. People with irresistible cravings get no other pleasure from eating than that of being freed from feeling poorly, caused by the reactive hypoglycemia. The eating is done out of necessity. The cravings for sweet foods are not caused by thoughts but by a physiological need. People dealing with reactive hypoglycemia can be thinking of something completely unrelated and all at once fall prey to an irresistible desire to eat. The gourmand continues to eat, even after he is no longer hungry, simply because it is tasty. The person suffering from reactive hypoglycemia stops eating once the feelings of discomfort are gone. Furthermore, he is only interested in sweet foods; the gourmand enjoys all foods.

🖐 Good to Know

The irresistible hungers of hypoglycemia should not be confused with the compulsive eating of bulimia. The bulimic is psychologically driven to eat from fear of a lack, and not when the absence of food is actually occurring, as is the case for the person experiencing hypoglycemia. Furthermore, the bulimic does not stop eating after the hunger has been sated, but continues to binge well beyond that point.

PHYSICAL DISORDERS

The extreme absence of sugar during attacks of reactive hypoglycemia can bring about a variety of physical ailments. Fatigue and a lack of energy are much more intense than in the case of simple hypoglycemia. The sense of fatigue is proportionate to the reactive state of the pancreas. The individual feels so weak that all momentum and enthusiasm are lacking. In serious cases the individual feels incapable of undertaking any task and even less able to deal with obstacles. Everything turns into a huge problem for this individual. Life stops seeming rosy and turns gray or even black.

The lack of sugar disrupts the functioning of the organs. Because the heart requires sugar to function properly, its absence prevents it from working normally. Blood pressure can drop to a varying degree depending on the person. It can be a minor case of low blood pressure with some slight dizziness, or, in more serious cases, there may be a major plunge of blood pressure along with dizzy spells. The person may even stagger and faint. Sometimes there is ringing in the ears or headaches. To restore the pressure to its normal level, the heart will suddenly accelerate its beat. Palpitations can result from this, panicking the individual.

The lungs are driven by the muscles. In the event of a lack of sugar, respiratory amplitude is reduced and consequently the intake of oxygen is also diminished. In mild cases the subject will only experience shortness of breath, sigh repeatedly, or yawn from the lack of air. In more serious cases the subject has the impression of suffocating and tries desperately to breathe. In this case the individual becomes nervous, or very anxious and panicked, precipitating heavy perspiration and hot flashes or cold sweat. Tingling sensations or pins and needles may cause unpleasant feelings in different areas of the body. The person becomes more or less hypersensitive to noises, odors, and light. The state of stress the person experiences can cause muscles to jerk uncontrollably or spasm. In this latter case, cramps and agonizing muscle pains will appear.

MENTAL DISORDERS

Before launching into the mental disorders created by reactive hypoglycemia, let's take a look at how the lack of sugar can affect the mind.

The headquarters for our mental life is the brain. Our thoughts, our feelings, our emotions, our way of looking at reality and reacting to it, our capacity for attention, concentration, learning, and memory are all dependent on how the brain functions. There is not a single reflection, reasoning, or emotion that can take place without it.

Now, the brain depends entirely on glucose to function properly. The brain is also exceptionally gluttonous for this substance. Although the brain represents only 2 percent of the body, it uses more glucose than any other organ. The body in its entirety needs around 200 grams of glucose a day. Out of these 200 grams, the brain uses two-thirds. When it is subjected to an extremely absorbing activity (e.g., intense intellectual labor, stress), its need for glucose increases even more.

Contrary to many other organs, the brain is unable to convert fat into glucose. It is therefore entirely dependent on the glucose that the bloodstream delivers to it. Nor is it capable of storing glucose, and its capacity for glucose in its tissues is quite small. Without an external supply, what it has on hand would allow it to continue functioning for only ten minutes.

All episodes of hypoglycemia, therefore, have negative repercussions on brain function. The more pronounced the reactive hypoglycemia, the greater the disruptions that it causes. As our entire mental life is dependent on the functioning of the brain, it is critical that it receive sufficient glucose.

The changes of the mental life observed in those suffering from episodes of reactive hypoglycemia can take place on two levels.

Cognitive Disorders

These troubles can span a wide range, from a simple lack of concentration or difficulty making decisions to mental confusion and false perceptions.

Emotional Disorders

These difficulties can range from simple impatience and irritability to fits of anger and even violence. They can manifest in the form of mental lethargy and a lack of zest for life, but they can also appear as attacks of anxiety without any cause, relentless worries, fears, phobias, weeping fits, and depressive states. A lack of inner assurance and emotional hypersensitivity may also be seen.

While each of these symptoms is bad enough to experience individually, for the reactive hypoglycemic the combination of several of them together can be sheer torture. Reactive hypoglycemia sufferers don't usually experience them all at the same time, but some at one time and others at another. They are therefore prey to a full variety of uncomfortable mental states over the course of each day.

The mental malaise that these individuals feel is all the more painful to experience as they usually do not know why this is happening to them. It remains incomprehensible because there are no external causes. Furthermore, no effort of will on their part allows them to change their condition, nor does the taking of any medicines. They have the impression that they are doomed to suffer this discomfort with no possibility of escaping it.

A similar malaise to that of people strongly affected by reactive hypoglycemia will also appear during insulin shock. When a diabetic receives a dose of insulin that is too high, it can cause a state of shock—with anxiety, cold sweats, trembling, dizzy spells—that even leads to losing consciousness. This state is known to be extremely unpleasant and stressful. But what the diabetic experiences only one time by accident, the individual afflicted with strong reactive hypoglycemia will live through repeatedly over the course of the day, every day.

When the mental and emotional disruptions are strong, those suffering from reactive hypoglycemia sometimes assume antisocial behaviors. Unable to control themselves or the situations confronting them, they have a tendency to seek isolation. They can become ferocious, wild, solitary, or even aggressive, quarrelsome, disrespectful, and rude, disrupting their lives with their spouses, families, and work colleagues.

All of these problems will continue as long as the necessary treatment is not established. This treatment quite simply consists of getting rid of the attacks of reactive hypoglycemia by replacing the bad sugars with good sugars. This is because, we should recall, if such an individual is suffering, it is not due to attack by a disease from the outside, but because of a poor choice of carbohydrate foods that put the body out of whack.

⚠ Caution!

If someone stricken by reactive hypoglycemia does not get adequate treatment with a change in diet, it is generally not out of unwillingness but out of ignorance. It is not widely known that mood disorders can be caused by insufficient sugar. Most often the problem is attributed to all sorts of other causes—anything but reactive hypoglycemia.

Dependency

The term *dependency* is customarily used for hard drugs (heroin, cocaine) or milder substances (alcohol, tobacco). However, a dependency on refined sugar is also possible. This comparison between refined sugar and drugs might seem a little daring because refined sugar is not a drug per se. However, the process of habituation and dependency are similar. Before showing how dependency on refined sugar gets established, let's take a general look at the process that creates addiction. I will use the example of alcohol as an illustration.

Mechanisms of Dependency

Someone who is stressed, frustrated, or sad turns to alcohol in an effort to drive away uncomfortable feelings. Because the person feels happier with the effect of the alcohol, it seems only natural to turn to it again on other occasions. If this individual does not pay attention, the consumption of alcohol can become more regular and increase in quantity, becoming detrimental. Alcohol's harmful effects are felt both physically and mentally. Mood changes occur because alcohol "burns away" many nutrients. It is therefore stealing them from the body, most particularly the brain and the nervous system, the chief supports of mental and emotional health. For example, a deficiency of magnesium can make a person, depending on the scope of the deficit, impatient, irritable, aggressive, or terribly violent.

The mood changes caused by alcohol are unpleasant. To get rid of them, the person turns again to alcohol, knowing from experience that it can provide relief. From this time forward, alcohol is no longer used to soothe the discomfort caused by external events (stress, problems, frustrations), but the bad feelings caused by the harmful effects of the alcohol itself. In other words, the substance that created the discomfort is also used to relieve it. A vicious cycle is created. Each time the person resorts to alcohol, it creates feelings of discomfort that push the individual to consume more alcohol. Convinced that alcohol is the only thing that can provide relief, the individual feels constantly compelled to turn to it again and again.

Avoiding alcohol consumption causes this person intense distress. There is an irresistible, urgent need to have another drink. The person cannot do without alcohol and is convinced it is the only way to feel good. In other words, the person is dependent.

> **Definition of dependency:** State resulting from the repeated consumption of an active mood-altering substance, characterized by the need to continue taking the substance and increasing the doses.
>
> *LE PETIT ROBERT* FRENCH DICTIONARY

The difference between sugar and drugs is that drugs have a mood-altering effect the first time they are taken, whereas refined sugar does not do so until the system has been disrupted.

Everything I just said about alcohol can be repeated with respect to refined white sugar.

The Case of Refined White Sugar

Following a conflict in the workplace, a person decides to eat a pastry for consolation and to restore a semblance of joy in life. Given the beneficial effects that are felt upon consumption, this individual will employ the same means to get comfort on other occasions. Over time the consumption of pastries increases, and the detrimental effects of bad sugars make themselves known. The pancreas becomes hyperreactive, and the person is in an ongoing state of reactive hypoglycemia on a regular basis, suffering from feelings of anxiety and malaise. The vicious cycle described for alcohol also establishes itself here. The person regularly consumes sugar to be free of the unpleasant and harmful effects of bad sugars, and thus becomes addicted to them.

Comparing a person under the influence of refined sugar to a drug addict is no exaggeration because of the many parallels existing between them.

A drug addict is regularly in a state of lack and feels a strong need to consume the drug of choice in order to feel good again. The same thing is true for the hypoglycemic with sugar. The person suffers repeatedly from a deficit in sugar that creates an irresistible craving. In both cases, the taking of the missing substance gives relief, but only for the short term. It needs to constantly be consumed again, with the result being that the lacks and demands control their lives.

If addicts are deprived of their drugs for a long time, they will feel increasingly bad and start to experience withdrawal symptoms. Just like a drug addict taking more and more of the drug and needing it more and more, the more the hypoglycemic consumes bad sugars, the more there will be cravings for sugar.

The major difference between the drug addict and the hypoglycemic is that it is quite difficult for the addict to quit taking the drug but relatively easy for the hypoglycemic to get free of a dependency on sugar.

TEST YOURSELF FOR REACTIVE HYPOGLYCEMIA

Diet and Symptoms Questionnaires

How can we know if we are suffering from reactive hypoglycemia?

THE DIET TEST

Reactive hypoglycemia only affects people who regularly eat high quantities of bad sugars. Is this your situation? To determine if it is, you'll need to scrutinize your diet. The questionnaire that follows seeks to provide evidence of whether you eat good or bad sugars. Answer the questions with a yes or no by checking off the box in the appropriate column.

	Yes	No
1. I put jam or another sweet spread on my toast.	☐	☐
2. I put refined sugar in my tea or coffee.	☐	☐
3. I like breakfasts that consist of pastries.	☐	☐
4. I eat white bread for breakfast.	☐	☐
5. My breakfast cereal is "frosted."	☐	☐
6. I add refined sugar to my breakfast cereal.	☐	☐

	Yes	No
7. When I feel hungry, I eat sweetened chocolate or cookies.	☐	☐
8. The pasta and grains (rice, couscous, etc.) I eat are refined.	☐	☐
9. I finish my meals with a sweet dessert.	☐	☐
10. I need a snack at ten o'clock and four o'clock, and these snacks are sweet (candy bars, cookies).	☐	☐
11. I like cola and other soft drinks.	☐	☐
12. I drink fruit juice with sugar added.	☐	☐
13. I prefer flavored yogurts (hence, sugar added).	☐	☐
14. If I eat cookies, they are made from refined white flour.	☐	☐
15. I prefer frosted or chocolate-covered cookies to plain ones.	☐	☐
16. I always carry chocolate or candy with me in case I suddenly feel tired.	☐	☐
17. I have a tendency to add sugar to my desserts.	☐	☐
18. I regularly eat refined white flour pasta and pizza.	☐	☐
19. I regularly drink sweet wines or cocktails.	☐	☐
20. I usually give in to my desire for a chocolate bar or ice cream, rather than eating fruit.	☐	☐

Add up the total of your answers.

Yes: _____

No: _____

Interpretation of the Results

15–20 "Yes" answers: You are a bad sugar champion. It is urgent that you change the way you eat.

10–15 "Yes" answers: You are a major consumer of bad sugars. Reforming your daily diet in this respect is essential.

5–10 "Yes" answers: You are a moderate consumer of bad sugars, but eating less of them will do you a world of good.

0–5 "Yes" answers: Bad sugars are not a problem for you.

This test is not sufficient on its own. It should be followed with a test that looks at whether or not you have symptoms of reactive hypoglycemia.

THE SYMPTOMS TEST

The "scientific" way to know if a person has problems with reactive hypoglycemia is to perform a test that triggers hyperglycemia. This test is long (it takes five to six hours) and requires regular taking of blood to measure the blood sugar level. It is also irritating and burdensome for the patient, so it is hardly ever used, for all of these reasons. A test in the form of a questionnaire is vastly preferred. This test was established by John F. Bumpus, a surgeon from Denver, Colorado, then expanded by Alan H. Nittler, M.D.*

The test consists of forty-six questions. Indicate the degree of the seriousness of your symptoms by choosing a number rating for each:

0 = no symptoms
1 = slight, rare symptoms
2 = moderate and occasional symptoms
3 = severe and common symptoms

When the questionnaire is complete, add up the numbers for each answer.

---

*For more information see *A New Breed of Doctor* (Pyramid House, 1972).

1. I have unusual cravings for sugar. ____
2. I get headaches in the afternoon. ____
3. I drink alcohol. ____
4. I have allergies, am prone to asthma attacks, have hay fever, or get skin rashes. ____
5. I wake up after a few hours of sleep. ____
6. I realize that I breathe with difficulty. ____
7. I have bad dreams. ____
8. My gums bleed. ____
9. I have blurred vision. ____
10. I have brown spots or patches on my skin. ____
11. I always get bruises, even when I bump into something lightly. ____
12. I have butterflies in my stomach, and cramps. ____
13. I have a hard time making up my mind. ____
14. I cannot get started on my day until I have a cup of coffee. ____
15. I cannot work under pressure. ____
16. I am constantly tired. ____
17. I am constantly exhausted. ____
18. I have convulsions. ____
19. I have strong cravings for candy or coffee in the afternoon. ____
20. I easily weep for no reason. ____
21. I am depressed. ____
22. I get dizzy spells. ____
23. I drink ____ cup(s) of coffee a day.
24. I must eat often, otherwise I have stomach cramps or weak spells. ____
25. I eat when I get nervous. ____
26. If meals are late, I feel weak. ____
27. When I eat, my weariness seems to vanish. ____
28. I am fearful. ____
29. When I am hungry, I begin shivering. ____
30. I have hallucinations. ____

31. My hands shake. ____
32. My heart starts beating fast if I skip a meal or do not eat early enough. ____
33. I am very emotional. ____
34. I get hungry between meals. ____
35. I have insomnia. ____
36. I feel uneasy or shaky within. ____
37. I am irritable before meals. ____
38. I lack energy. ____
39. I make mountains out of molehills. ____
40. I have the blues; I am melancholy and always look at the dark side. ____
41. I have a poor memory. ____
42. I have difficulty taking the initiative. ____
43. I feel somnolent after meals. ____
44. I fall asleep during the day. ____
45. I feel weak, as if I have no strength. ____
46. I am alarmed, anxious, and constantly worried. ____

Total: _____

Interpretation of the Results

If your total comes out higher than 25, you are subject to attacks of reactive hypoglycemia, especially if you answered with the number 3 (severe and common symptoms) to three of the eight questions numbered below:

16	17	24	26	27	29	43	44
☐	☐	☐	☐	☐	☐	☐	☐

If the result of your test indicates that you are subject to reactive hypoglycemia, it is imperative that you remove bad sugar from your diet.

THE GLYCEMIC INDEX

Food Rankings and Their Effect on Blood Sugar Levels

To determine the identity of the bad sugars, scientists have studied another criterion in addition to that of unadulterated carbohydrate foods used in holistic healing. In the early 1980s, Canadian researcher David Jenkins led the first team to define and explore criteria for a glycemic index (GI) that measures how specific foods affect blood sugar.

DETERMINING THE GLYCEMIC INDEX

The glycemic index makes it possible to precisely quantify each food's ability to raise blood sugar level. The higher the figure in this index, the greater the food's ability to trigger a considerable spike in the content of sugar in the blood, and the reverse. The glycemic index of foods is established through comparison to a food used as a reference, in this instance, pure glucose, which creates the highest spike in blood sugar level that we know. Glucose has been given the highest reading on a measuring scale that goes from 1 to 100. It has therefore been given the GI of 100.

By measuring the rise in blood sugar level caused by each food and comparing it to the benchmark element, glucose, each food can be given its own GI. The closer the glycemic index of a food is to 100, the greater the hyperglycemic effect of the food, and the greater the release of insulin. On the other hand, the lower the glycemic index, the less the food's ability to raise blood sugar levels to hyperglycemic levels, and the same for the corresponding release of insulin.

The measurement of the glycemic index of each food is made in the following way: Volunteers eat a portion of food containing the equivalent of 50 grams of glucose. As each food has a different carbohydrate content, the amount of each food ingested will vary. For example, a 600-gram portion of raw carrots has 50 grams of glucose, while 100 grams of whole grain bread is enough to provide the same amount of glucose.

The effect on blood sugar level is then measured every thirty minutes for a period of three hours. The results are then compared with that of the glucose, and the glycemic index is established based on these findings.

RANKING FOODS

As the GI is drawn up numerically, it is possible to establish a hierarchy of foods based on their glycemic index ranking. This list can begin with the foods that have the lowest GI rankings, or the reverse. To facilitate use of the results, this list is next divided into three groups based on whether the glycemic index level of the food is low, medium, or high, and then drawn up in a chart.

In our first group we find foods with a low glycemic index ranking, which means their level is 35 and below. In the second we find foods with a mid-range GI, with readings above 35 and up to 50. In the third are those with a high GI, which are all the foods 55 and above. (All index numbers are rounded to the nearest multiple of 5.)

FOODS AND PRODUCTS WITH A LOW GI

Dried apricots	35	Mung beans	25
Oranges, peaches, nectarines, apples, plums (fresh fruits)	35	Green lentils	25
Celery root (raw)	35	Whole almond paste (sugar free)	25
Figs (fresh)	35	Dark chocolate (>70 percent cocoa)	25
White or red beans	35	Dark chocolate (>85 percent cocoa)	20
Tomato juice	35	Powdered cocoa (no sugar added)	20
Flax, sesame, poppy, sunflower (seeds)	35	Artichoke, eggplant, hearts of palm (fresh)	20
Essene bread (from sprouted grains)	35	Lemon (fresh or juice with no added sugar)	20
Green peas (fresh)	35	Ratatouille	20
Chickpeas (canned)	35	Soy yogurt (plain)	20
Applesauce (unsweetened)	35	Agave (syrup)	15
Quinoa	35	Almonds, hazelnuts, walnuts, cashews, soy nuts	15
Yogurt (plain)	35	Almond flour	15
Wild rice	35	Asparagus, chard, celery, leeks	15
Soy yogurt (flavored, sweetened)	35	Sauerkraut, cauliflower, cabbage, Brussels sprouts, broccoli	15
Coconut flour	35	Peppers, mushroom, zucchini, cucumber	15
Apricot, grapefruit, pear (fruit)	30	Peanuts, pine nuts, pistachios	15
Garlic	30	Shallots, ginger, onions, olives	15
Beets, carrots (raw), green beans	30	Endive, chicory, spinach, salad greens	15
Cottage cheese (plain)	30	Navy beans, snow peas, flat beans	15
Cow's milk, almond, oat, soy milk	30	Tofu (soy)	15
Brown lentils, chickpeas	30	Avocado	10
Tomatoes	30	Spices (pepper, parsley, basil, oregano, caraway, cinnamon, vanilla, and so on)	5
Goji berries	25		
Cherries, raspberries, blackberries, strawberries, red currants	25		
Soy flour	25		
Flageolets, split peas	25		
Pumpkin seeds	25		

The provided GI tables, developed by nutrition researcher Michel Montignac, another GI pioneer of the 1980s, show the GI of the most common foods. Meat and fish are not listed as their glucose content, and thus their ability to cause hyperglycemia, is negligible.

FOODS AND PRODUCTS WITH A MEDIUM GI

Couscous, whole grain semolina	50	Green peas (canned)	45
Apple juice (no added sugar)	50	Grapes	45
Kiwi	50	Brown basmati rice	45
Muesli (no added sugar)	50	Tomato sauce, canned tomatoes	45
Sweet potato	50	Rye (flour or bread)	45
Whole grain pasta	50	Raw cider	40
White basmati rice	50	Fava beans (raw)	40
Whole brown rice	50	Dried figs	40
Surimi (fake crab)	50	Oat flakes (uncooked)	40
Pineapple	45	Oat flour	40
Banana (green)	45	Red beans (canned)	40
Whole bulgur wheat	45	Carrot juice (no added sugar)	40
Whole grains (no added sugar)	45	Whole grain bread (100 percent, with pure yeast)	40
Jam (no added sugar)	45	Prunes	40
Spelt (flour or wholegrain bread)	45	Sesame paste	40
Grapefruit juice (no added sugar)	45	Buckwheat, whole grain (bread or flour)	40
Orange juice (pressed, no added sugar)	45	Al dente white spaghetti	40
Coconut	45		

FOODS AND PRODUCTS WITH A HIGH GI

Glucose	100	Whole (unrefined) sugar	70
Glucose syrup	100	Jam (made with sugar)	65
Rice flour	95	Refined couscous, semolina	65
Potato starch	95	Chestnut flour	65
Maltodextrin	95	Fava beans (cooked)	65
Baked potatoes	95	Corn kernels	65
Instant potatoes	90	Standard muesli (sugar or honey added)	65
Sticky rice	90		
Cooked carrots	85	Pain au chocolat	65
Corn flakes	85	Rye bread (whole or half)	65
Refined white flour, bread, crackers	85	Steamed or boiled potatoes	65
		Raisins	65
Rice milk	85	Sorbet (average)	65
Cornstarch	85	Apricot in syrup	60
Minute rice	85	Banana (ripe)	60
Puffed rice, rice crackers	85	Chestnuts	60
Mashed potatoes	80	Ice cream (average)	60
Pumpkin	75	Melon	60
Chocolate bars (sugar added)	70	Honey	60
Wheat crackers	70	Cocoa powder (sweetened)	60
Cookies (average)	70	Long-grain aromatic rice	60
Brioche	70	Cooked bulgur	55
Refined sugar cereals	70	Grape juice	55
Chips	70	Ketchup	55
Colas, sodas, soft drinks	70	Mustard	55
Croissant	70	Nutella	55
Dates	70	White spaghetti (well-cooked)	55
Standard white rice	70		
Refined sugar (sucrose)	70	Maple syrup	55

By examining the tables we can see that the division of the three foods is basically the following:

FIRST GROUP:
FOODS WITH LOW GI

- The majority of fruits and vegetables
- Oleaginous foods
- Leguminous foods
- Dairy products
- Sprouted grains

SECOND GROUP:
FOODS WITH MEDIUM GI

- Whole grains
- Products made from whole grains: bread, pasta, crackers, and so on
- Fruit juices
- Several fresh and dried fruits that do not appear in the first group

THIRD GROUP:
FOODS WITH HIGH GI

- Refined white sugar and sweets
- All-purpose white flour and products made from it: bread, pasta, and so on
- Potatoes
- Chestnuts
- Several whole grains
- Several fruits and juices
- Honey
- Dates

A Little History

Glycemic index tables vary depending on a number of factors, and the current standard index shows different category breaks for low, medium, and high from those cited here, with high GI not starting until 70. Montignac explains that this is because we now have research that was not available when the GI system was originally proposed. In addition, he suggests that the standard accepted index accommodates food manufacturers desirous of selling more products, as well as nutritionists who are comfortable with their current level of knowledge and practice. It is recommended that readers consult several sources to help them determine their food choices.

WHY ARE THERE SUCH LARGE DIFFERENCES IN THE GI OF SIMILAR FOODS?

GI numbers take several different factors into consideration:

The Presence of Plant Fiber

Once they have been chewed, fruits travel through the intestines in the form of mash. The sugars from the fruit are surrounded there by plant fiber from the pulp of the fruit. The presence of the fibers reduces the sugars' contact with the walls of the intestines. This has the effect of slowing their penetration of the bloodstream, so the body's blood sugar level does not rise very high. For this reason, many fruits have a low glycemic index.

The process is different for fruit juices. Most juices are low in roughage because the bulk of the fibers remain in the juice extractors. For this reason the sugar in the juice makes direct contact with the intestinal walls and rapidly enters the bloodstream. A good deal of glucose enters the bloodstream, so the GI of fruit juices is therefore higher than that of fruits consumed whole with their peels.

For example, an apple has a GI of 30, but apple juice has a GI of 50; grapes have a GI of 45, while grape juice has a GI of 55. However, if whole fruit is liquefied in a powerful home machine, the juice retains the same GI as the whole fruit.

What was just said about the influence of fiber on the GI of fruits is also valid for grains. In its natural state, cereal grain is enveloped in a husk (pericarp) that is high in fiber. This is no longer the case once the grain has been refined. It is stripped of its husk for the purpose of obtaining a white grain (white rice, for example) or all-purpose white flour. People use the term *whole grain* when speaking of grains that are still in their natural state—still in possession of their fibrous husk—and *refined grain* when speaking of grains from which this fibrous husk has been removed.

The glucose provided by these two kinds of food enters the bloodstream in different ways. The glucose supplied by cereal grains enters the bloodstream slowly because of the presence of fibers. The blood sugar level does not climb very high. In any case, it is lower than when refined grains (all-purpose white flour, white bread, etc.) are consumed. The glucose provided by these latter products enters the bloodstream much more rapidly, which causes the blood sugar level to soar higher. This is easily shown by the index, on which the GI of whole grain bread is 65 whereas that of white bread is 85, and whole wheat flour has a GI of 45 versus all-purpose white flour at 85.

The Nature of Starch

There are two forms of starch:

- Amylose consists of chains of glucose whose molecules are organized in a complex way. Their structure makes them difficult for the digestive enzymes to break down into smaller pieces, so the glucose provided by amylose only becomes available to the body gradually. Its GI is low.
- Amylopectin also consists of long chains of glucose, but the molecules have a simple organization. Digestive enzymes break them down easily. The sugar in amylopectin is consequently speedily released into the bloodstream causing blood sugar levels to soar. Its GI is high.

Amylose and amylopectin are found in the composition of the starch of all foods, but the proportions in which they are found in these starches varies from one kind of food to another. Some starches consist of a large quantity of amylose but a small proportion of amylopectin, and some of just the opposite. The GI of a food will be either high or low depending on the proportion of these two components.

The starch in leguminous foods consists of 30 to 60 percent amylose. This, added to the fact that leguminous foods are high in fiber, gives them a low GI (30 for lentils and chickpeas). The starch of potatoes, on the other hand, is high in amylopectin. This component represents 80 percent of potato starch. The GI for potatoes is therefore high: 95 for baked potatoes and 80 for mashed potatoes.

The content of amylose and amylopectin in grains falls somewhere between that of leguminous foods and potatoes, so their GI ranks are also in between: 40 for whole buckwheat; 45 for rye, brown basmati rice, and spelt; 50 for brown rice; 60 for whole wheat flour.

📘 A Little History

Basmati rice is named for its sweet, exotic aroma; its name means "queen of fragrance" in Hindi. Although relatively new to the United States, basmati rice has been cultivated in India and Pakistan since at least 1766. Be sure to choose brown basmati rice (not white basmati).

Cooking

Cooking will alter the glycemic index in several ways.

On the one hand it softens the fiber of fruits and vegetables, which increases the bioavailability of the sugars contained in their pulp. This is why the GI of raw carrots is 30 but that of cooked carrots is 85. On the other hand, heat "predigests" starch, which means that the long chains of glucose are broken into smaller chains. This makes the glucose available to the body much more quickly.

The GI of a cooked grain is consequently higher than the GI of the same grain that has been partially cooked or is raw. Al dente spaghetti has a GI of 40 while well-cooked spaghetti has one of 55. Uncooked oat flakes have a GI of 40, while cooked oats have a rank of 60.

The influence of cooking on the glycemic index is given here as information only; this is not a recommendation to eat raw or undercooked foods that need to be cooked to be fully digestible.

Puffed Cereal Grains

Cereal grains have a very firm, perhaps even hard consistency. To make them softer and easier to chew, they can be puffed, as is the case with Rice Krispies, rice cakes, and certain crackers and snacks.

Grains are puffed by being deliberately cooked under pressure to a point at which this pressure is suddenly released. The wall of the grain bursts and the grain increases in size. The "explosion" that occurs in this deconcentrated grain aerates its internal structure. This makes it much easier for the digestive enzymes to transform it inside the body. The glucose is quickly freed and enters the bloodstream much more quickly than is the case with the entire whole grain. As a result, the GI of white rice is 70 while that of puffed white rice is 85. The GI of corn kernels is 65; however, that of popcorn is 85.

BAD SUGARS AS VIEWED FROM THE GI APPROACH

Based on this approach, the bad sugars are the foods whose sugars cause blood sugar levels to soar to very high levels, which thereby encourages the exhaustion of the pancreas, attacks of reactive hypoglycemia, and weight gain. We are therefore dealing with foods that rank high on the glycemic index, or to be more specific, those in the third group of the table provided earlier.

In this category we find all the foods that supply bad sugar as defined by the naturopathic approach. In fact, refined sugar and flour, as well as all the products manufactured from them, can be found in this third group. The naturopathic approach and that of the glycemic index are in complete agreement on this point.

They do differ, though, on another point. In the third group we also find foods that naturopathy identifies as being good sugars: various whole grains, certain fruits, potatoes, chestnuts, honey, and so forth. According to the GI approach, these are all bad sugars. Are these foods from nature truly bad?

The first observation that leaps to mind: these foods for the most part have a GI of 65 or lower but are still in the highest group in the Montignac system we are using. And while the GI number is based on an objective system of measurement (the varying rise in the blood sugar level), the division of the glycemic index into three groups (low, medium, and high) is based not on objective data but on the subjective evaluation of the person dividing the foods into the three groups.

The subjectivity at work in this division process is obvious if we examine the work of different authors. The one provided in the tables reproduced on pages 94–96 is the strictest classification (the Montignac system). It starts its list of high GI foods at 55. But there are other approaches that offer alternative ranges. They place the threshold of high GIs at 60 and 70.

DIVISION OF FOODS

	LOW GI	MEDIUM GI	HIGH GI
Montignac	0–35	40–50	55–100
Berthon	0–40	45–55	60–100
Houlbert	0–55	60–65	70–100

As we can see, there is disparity among the tables of these three researchers. If we hypothetically rank the bottommost level of foods in the high GI bracket as the average of the two higher estimates noted above (60 and 70), at 65, what do we see? Now the foods considered high GI—that is, 65 and higher—are almost all considered to be bad sugars (refined sugar and flour). Everybody is in agreement, therefore, that these substances are bad sugars.

Likewise, if 65 is the dividing line for foods that fall into the high GI group, as I just suggested, all the foods lower than 65 in this list then fall into the group of medium GI and out of the group of bad sugars. These include corn, boiled potatoes, raisins, ripe bananas, rye bread, and honey.

This is more in keeping with reality. In fact, while these foods certainly create a hyperglycemic state that triggers insulin release, they do not promote the reactive hypoglycemia that pushes the individual to eat sugary foods.

Furthermore, in practice people do not develop a craving for sweets after eating baked potatoes (GI 95), cooked carrots (GI 85), pumpkin soup (GI 80), or dates (GI 70). Sugar cravings do not normally follow ingestion of these foods. They cannot therefore be considered to be bad sugars. A person suffering from constant recurrences of reactive hypoglycemia and irrepressible cravings for sugar should not eliminate these natural foods with high GI rankings. For these people they are not as harmful as the GI system might lead them to believe.

THE GLYCEMIC INDEX AND WEIGHT GAIN

The GI system is still useful, however. It is quite important for people who are overweight and do not wish to gain any more pounds to understand and respect this index. The fact remains that food with a high GI triggers a rapid strike in blood glucose levels and a subsequent strong release of insulin. We know that when the glycogen reserves are full, insulin can no longer transform the glucose entering the bloodstream into this substance. Insulin then converts this glucose into fat, which is stored in the tissues. With each new intake of carbohydrates, another addition to the fat reserves in the tissues takes place.

Over time this process contributes to weight gain, then obesity.

To avoid storing glucose in the form of fat, top priority is to avoid consuming foods that trigger the release of large amounts of insulin. All these foods are found in the high GI group.

Consequently, the GI tables are most useful for people with weight problems. They can avoid gaining more weight by choosing to mainly eat foods with low GIs and eating those with medium GIs with greater restraint. As for the foods found in the high GI group, those that are bad sugars should be totally eliminated (refined sugar, all-purpose flour, sweets, cookies, and so forth). Foods that are "healthful" and have "good sugars," such as potatoes and dates, should be consumed with moderation.

The recommendations given here for controlling weight are derived from the GI system. Other measures (stimulation of the liver, exercise) should also be applied to obtain good results.

PRACTICAL GUIDELINES FOR REACTIVE HYPOGLYCEMIA SUFFERERS

People wishing to avoid attacks of reactive hypoglycemia and the sugar dependency it creates (as well as diabetics, borderline diabetics, and anyone with a genetic predisposition to diabetes) don't need to consult a GI table to decide whether or not they can eat a particular food. All they need to do is avoid the bad sugars as they are defined in naturopathy (refined sugar, sweets, refined all-purpose flour, and refined cereal grains and products). It is easy to identify these products as they are all man-made.

This way of approaching things is simpler than constantly checking tables.

PART 2

A Practical Guide to Replacing Bad Sugars with Good Sugars

Once they have become aware of the adverse effects of bad sugars, many people feel the need to reform their diets. But what do they need to do to proceed correctly? What factors need to be considered? What foods or sugars should be eliminated? With what should they be replaced? How strict must they be?

The purpose of the second part of this book is to answer all these questions. Each chapter presents one important aspect of this dietary overhaul and explains the practical means of realizing it. Tables are also provided that make it easy to find the most crucial information, as well as advice for implementing a more healthful way of eating.

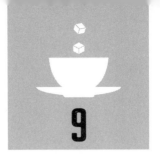

9

IDENTIFYING AND ELIMINATING BAD SUGARS

Goal: Learn to recognize the different kinds of bad sugars and identify the ones you are eating.

Because bad sugars are actually harmful to your health, they need to be replaced with good sugars.

In chapter 2 we looked at the bad sugars and why they are harmful, but you may find the summary lists that follow useful, starting with refined sugar and foods that are high in this substance. We will then proceed the same way with refined grains.

As for foods with good sugars that we must eat to replace these bad sugars, they will be the subject of the next chapter.

LIST OF REFINED SUGARS

This list includes all the refined sugars, whether they are white or a varying shade of brown, regardless of whether this brown color was obtained by the addition of dyes or the refining process was not carried to the final stages. This list also includes all the refined sugars whose chemical structure was altered to give them a soft consistency. What all these sugars have in common is that they do not contain any vitamins or minerals, or if they do it is in such negligible quantities that they have no health benefits. It is therefore recommended that you eliminate them from your diet.

- Raw sugar (organic sugar)
- Turbinado sugar
- Brown sugar (light, golden brown, dark)
- Plantation sugar
- Granulated white table sugar
- Confectioners' sugar
- Invert sugar
- Sugar in large crystals
- Liquid sugar
- Corn syrup
- High-fructose corn syrup
- Glucose syrup
- Rock candy
- Table molasses
- Fructose
- Dextrose
- Xylitol (Birch syrup)

LIST OF FOODS HIGH IN REFINED SUGAR

Refined sugar can be found in substantial proportions in a number of foods. The sugar content can range from partial (sweetened yogurt is from 10 to 12 percent sugar; with sweetened fruit added it's around 14 to 20 percent) to almost total (candy is 99 percent).

SWEETS

- Candies
- Sweetened chewing gums
- Sweetened fruit snacks
- Stewed fruit
- Candied chestnuts
- Sweetened chocolate
- Marzipan
- Chocolate bars
- Sweetened cereal bars
- Sweetened nut bars

BREAKFAST FOODS

- Jams and jellies
- Sweetened spreads such as Nutella
- Table molasses
- Breakfast cereals with sugar added
- Breakfast cereals with chocolate

SNACK FOODS

- Cookies made with sugar
- Cakes
- Sweet rolls
- Doughnuts
- Pastries
- Dates or prunes in syrup
- Sweetened yogurt

DESSERTS

- Ice cream
- Sweet custard
- Caramel flan

- Sweetened creams
- Sweetened fruit tarts
- Compotes with sugar

BEVERAGES

- Commercial soft drinks
- Stimulating sport beverages with caffeine
- Fruit juice with added sugar
- Chocolate beverages
- Malted beverages
- Sodas
- Tea, coffee, herbal tea with sugar added
- Liqueurs
- Cordials
- Cocktails sweetened with sugar or syrup

The sugar content of commercial soft drinks is around 9 teaspoons per 12-ounce can. Average annual consumption per person in the United States, though falling, is still around 39 gallons annually per person, or around 416 cans, equaling 3,744 teaspoons of sugar. That is a lot of sugar!

⚠ Caution!

You are unlikely to see 9 teaspoons of sugar listed on a soft drink or food label. However, any time you see any variation of corn syrup or glucose syrup, be aware that it is a code name for sugar.

Because the harmful effects of sugar are becoming much more well-known, some candies, desserts, soft drinks, and so forth are no longer manufactured with refined sugar but use artificial sweeteners. All sweet foods that are produced for diabetics are also sweetened artificially. However, artificial sweeteners are also generally considered to be harmful to health.

FOODS WITH HIDDEN SUGARS

The sweet flavor of many foods lets us know immediately if they contain sugar. On the other hand, there are foods that contain added sugar that cannot be detected by taste because only small quantities of sugar are present, or because its flavor is hidden by other, more potent flavors.

This includes, for example, salty foods to which a little sugar has been added (most often refined sugar) to give them a particular flavor. For example, soups, gravies, and marinades are salted, but often food product manufacturers attempt to make them taste more interesting by adding a little sugar. No sweet taste betrays the presence of this sugar in sauces and soups, so no one realizes these foods contain it. For this reason, this sugar is described as "hidden sugar." When you eat a food with sugar concealed in it, you do not even realize you are eating any sugar.

Hidden sugar is also present in foods with a sweet flavor, such as sweetened fruit juices, flavored yogurt, and breakfast cereals that have dried fruits and other items mixed into them. This sugar has been added to make them more appealing. Because people expect a certain food to taste sweet, they do not notice that sugar has been added. This added sugar is concealed by the already sweet taste of the food, and it turns a healthful food into something that is not.

Hidden sugar is found in varying quantities in different foods. Added together, these small quantities of sugar end up representing a relatively appreciable quantity.

FOODS WITH HIDDEN SUGAR

- Sausage, sweet or spicy
- Cold cuts
- Hamburger
- Prepared dishes (such as lasagna)
- Gnocchi
- Pizza dough
- Soup
- Ketchup
- Salad dressing
- Grilling sauces
- Barbecue sauce
- Tomato sauce
- Mayonnaise
- Mustard
- Salty crackers
- Dry breakfast cereals
- Bread products, especially pastries and doughnuts
- Condiments
- Flavored yogurt
- Soda

To know whether a food contains hidden sugar, make it a habit to read the ingredients label on the package.

LIST OF REFINED GRAINS

Refined grains are consumed in the form of processed breakfast cereals as well as refined flours and all the many food products made from them.

BREAKFAST GRAINS

- Cereal grains (white rice, white or pearl barley, refined rye and sorghum, quick oats, and so on)
- Cereal flakes (cornflakes and so on)
- Puffed grains (crisped rice, sugary puffs, etc.)
- Novelty shapes (o's, loops, crunch mixtures, and so on)

Flours

The label or packaging of a flour will always give an indication of its characteristics. All flour that is not whole grain or a blend that includes whole grain is refined and consequently consists of bad sugars. Whatever grain they were produced from, you should avoid refined flour.

THE MOST COMMON REFINED FLOURS

- All-purpose white flour
- Cake flour
- White rice flour
- White rye flour

FOODS HIGH IN REFINED WHITE FLOUR

BAKED GOODS

- Bread made from all-purpose white flour or refined flour blend
- Crackers, crisp breads, zwieback, and so on, made from all-purpose white flour
- Breakfast breads, croissant, brioche, Danish pastry, rolls, muffins, scones, cakes

PASTA AND DOUGH

- Spaghetti, noodles, and other types of pasta made from all-purpose white flour
- Ravioli, lasagna, tortellini, and so on made from refined white flour
- Pizza dough made from all-purpose flour

VARIOUS FOODS

- Cookies made from all-purpose flour
- Crepes and pancakes made from all-purpose flour
- Cake made from all-purpose or cake flour
- Granola bars made from refined grains

For the sake of simplification, the lists I have compiled are those foods that are made with either refined sugars or refined grains. There are many foods or food preparations, though, that combine both kinds of bad sugars. For example, cookies are made from both all-purpose flour and refined sugar. Pastries and other breakfast breads are another example, as well as sugary breakfast cereals. Because they combine the harmful effects offered by both kinds of bad sugar, these foods should be eliminated from your diet.

IDENTIFYING BAD SUGARS IN YOUR DIET

Once we know which foods contain the bad sugars, we can look for which of those sugars are present in our own daily diet. An indispensable tool for performing this research is the evaluation of a standard menu—a menu that is representational of what we eat on a daily basis.

Establishing a Standard Menu

Nobody eats the same thing every day. Most often, the composition of our meals varies from one day to the next. However, despite how varied these meals might seem, certain constant themes appear. The main meals can be broken down to two or three variations. In fact, in a meal composed of a protein, a starch, and a vegetable, the fact that the protein might be veal, beef, or chicken does not fundamentally change the composition of the meal. It involves a kind of meat, as opposed to another protein food such as cheese or eggs.

It is possible to identify a standard menu by bringing such considerations into awareness. It is a good idea to write it down because this will ensure that these characteristics emerge more clearly.

Jot down everything you eat and drink from when you get up in the morning until you go to bed at night: on waking, breakfast (don't forget to include the tea or coffee), mid-morning snack, lunch (including any bread you eat with it), afternoon tea or snack, dinner (and dessert!), and drinks or foods consumed after dinner. Some people will also need to be sure to include everything they munch on between meals (various sweets, cookies, nuts, candies, chips, sweetened coffee drinks).

In the fictional menu example provided on the facing page, the different variations on a particular meal are separated by an "or." There is no need to go into extensive detail when there is no call to do so. For example, "cooked vegetables" or "raw vegetables" is sufficient. On the other hand, "drink," "grain," or "dessert" is too vague. It has to be specified whether or not the dessert is made with refined or whole sugar, and if the grain is whole or not.

Examples of the Standard Menu

Once the standard menu has been drawn up, underline all the foods containing bad sugars. This is demonstrated in the example below:

6:30 a.m.	coffee + white sugar
7:00 a.m.	white bread/bagel/English muffin (two slices or halves) + butter + jelly + two coffees with milk/cream + sugar
9:00 a.m.	one tea/coffee + milk/cream + sugar + sweetened cold cereal + milk *or* one tea/coffee + cream + sugar + piece of sweetened chocolate
12:00 p.m.	meat with sauce + French fries + vegetable + white bread + one cookie *or* sandwich (white bread) with ham + yogurt with fruit and sugar + salad *or* fish + brown basmati rice + raw vegetables + fresh fruit
Drink	6-ounce glass of wine or 10-ounce bottle of soda
4:00 p.m.	semi-dark bread + one chocolate bar + one coffee + cream + sugar *or* one pastry + coffee + sugar *or* one sweet bread + one hot chocolate
7:00 p.m.	cold cuts + sourdough roll *or* grilled meat + French fries + chocolate pudding *or* white flour fruit tart + whipped cream
Drink	herb tea with sugar *or* glass of sweetened fruit juice
9:00 p.m.	cookies with chocolate + can of soda

Analysis of the Standard Menu

If you have only underlined two or three food items in your daily menu, then your consumption of bad sugars is low.

In the opposite case, you are eating an unhealthy amount of sugar and these are foods that should be eliminated from your diet and replaced with good sugars.

HOW STRICT MUST YOU BE?

The question has a different answer depending on whether you are healthy or sick.

Of course it is in the best interest of those enjoying good health to eliminate bad sugars if they want to remain healthy. There is no crying urgency for them to do so, however, given the fact that the quantity they are eating is not enough to make them ill. Their elimination does not need to be too strict or intensive. A gradual transition will be sufficient.

For those who are ill, the elimination must be strict and speedy.

Individuals who are suffering from reactive hypoglycemia in particular must be very rigorous in their elimination of bad sugars. In such a case the pancreas is reacting very swiftly to the ingestion of these bad sugars. If someone eliminates most of them but still keeps eating a few, it will continue to overreact and trigger attacks of reactive hypoglycemia. If every single one of them is removed from the diet, the pancreas will unlearn its bad habit and learn how to function normally again more quickly. That said, the elimination of refined white sugar and sweets is more important than that of refined all-purpose flour.

The other patients who must strictly eliminate bad sugars from their diets are diabetics. In such cases the pancreas has already been exhausted by bad sugars and is further weakened by continued consumption.

How should people who are not as drastically affected—those whose consumption of bad sugars has led them to suffer from less dramatic illnesses; for example, eczema, bronchitis, rheumatism, and so forth—proceed? At first glance, it would seem possible to be more lenient about removing bad sugar from the diet, but pursuing this course would only be to their detriment. These diseases can only be cured by removing their cause, which in this case means eliminating bad sugars. By not taking this step, the cure will be only partially successful, or take longer to achieve, if it is ever achieved at all. So in these cases, too, it is simply better to remove all the bad sugars from the diet.

Once cured of these diseases, the person should definitely avoid going back to a diet containing bad sugars, or the same health disorders will soon reappear. Once you have adopted new and good habits, you should keep them.

IS COMPLETE ELIMINATION POSSIBLE?

Is the body capable of functioning without any refined sugar and flour? Total elimination is entirely possible. In fact, the body can do perfectly well without the bad sugars, for it can find all the good sugars it needs in the foods provided by nature. Proof for this can be seen in the fact that the human body functioned perfectly well without bad sugars until about two hundred years ago.

There are, however, a few good reasons to be more flexible in the application of this principle in certain cases.

The first reason is that there are some individuals who are not capable of properly digesting culinary preparations made with good sugars, such as whole grains and dried fruits, and eating them causes a stomachache. Food that is not digested properly produces considerable toxins, which trigger diseases or cause their reappearance. In these cases, then, it is a far better idea to consume ingredients that are a little less hearty; for example (and surprisingly!), all-purpose white flour. Of course, there will be a lack of nutrients, but the production of toxins will be lower. The individual can metabolize them better, and the final health result is better.

Whole sugar, on the other hand, is easy to digest, so there is no reason to replace it with any sugar that is not complete.

WHY WE CONTINUE TO EAT BAD SUGARS

For some people, bad sugars continue to be tolerated for psychological reasons. Perhaps they feel a great desire to follow a strict diet that completely eliminates bad sugars but cannot carry it through for lack of will or perseverance. When they become disappointed by their failure to be entirely strict, they drop all efforts and fall back into old habits. In such cases it is advisable not to set sights too high at the start. Eating half the accustomed amount of sweets, or eating white rice at one out of two meals, and so forth may not be very strict, but it is a step in the right direction. Over time, new habits will get established, and the need for bad sugars will decrease.

Other people are fully aware that these sugars are bad for them, but they have a great desire to eat some dessert or other sweet thing that they loved to eat in the past. If they try to go cold turkey on this food, their desire can turn into an obsession. In this case an occasional lapse can be justified to "take the edge off" the craving. This lapse is also justified for family celebrations, anniversaries, or work gatherings in order not to cause social friction. Eating something made with bad sugar from time to time when your diet is otherwise healthy does not lend itself to adverse consequences, as long as these lapses remain exceptions.

With practice the need for these little lapses diminishes over time. Someone who has grown accustomed to eating mostly good sugars will experience less and less desire to eat bad ones; pastries, chocolate, and commercial soft drinks will be too sweet for their palates. When they taste them again, they probably will not like them very much. They may even seem sickeningly sweet and therefore even less of a temptation. However, the memory of how a food formerly tasted can keep someone emotionally attached to a certain bad sugar, and even after it stops tasting good, it may be sought out in an effort to re-create the pleasure it once brought.

If "bad sugars summon more bad sugars," as we saw earlier, the corollary for this is that "good sugars drive bad sugars away." In other words, the more we eat the good sugars offered by nature, the less we want to eat the bad sugars.

The body needs to receive fuel in the form of sugar to function properly. Eliminating bad sugars from your diet is consequently only half of the solution. They need to be replaced with good sugars.

EATING GOOD SUGARS—
OPTIONS AND REPLACEMENTS

Goal: Continue eating the foods with good sugars that are already part of your diet, but replace any bad sugars you're eating with good sugars.

The body needs good sugars to function properly. In order to enjoy good health or to recover it when you are ill, it is therefore necessary to eat foods that contain them, including the foods you are already eating. You must also replace the bad sugars in your daily diet with good ones.

WHY WE NEED FOODS WITH GOOD SUGARS

Whole foods with good sugars are beneficial for our health. They are healthy because:

- They give us the energy we need.
- They are not vitamin or mineral deficient.
- They produce few toxins.
- They do not cause reactive hypoglycemia.

List of Foods with Good Sugars

FRUIT

- Fresh fruits: apples, grapes, pears, and so on
- Berries: raspberries, strawberries, blackberries, and so on
- Citrus fruits: oranges, tangerines, grapefruit, and so on
- Dried fruits: raisins, figs, dates, and so on
- Fruit juices (no added sugar)

VEGETABLES

- Sweet vegetables: carrots, beets, sweet potatoes, onions, and so on
- The juice from these vegetables

STARCHY FOODS

- Potatoes
- Chestnuts

BEANS

- Soybeans
- Lentils
- White beans

WHOLE GRAINS

- Whole wheat
- Whole oats
- Whole rye
- Whole spelt
- Whole (husked) barley
- Whole (brown) rice
- Whole corn
- Whole millet

- Whole buckwheat
- Whole quinoa (technically a seed, but used as a grain)

WHOLE FLOURS

- Whole wheat flour
- White whole wheat flour*
- Whole oat flour
- Brown rice flour
- Almond flour
- Coconut flour
- Whole rye flour
- Whole corn flour

Whole grain flours can also be blended with other flours to still support health but produce lighter—and, for some, more palatable—grain-based foods.

WHOLE GRAIN BREADS, CRACKERS, COOKIES, AND PASTA

- Whole grain bread
- Whole grain crackers
- Whole grain cookies
- Whole grain pasta
- Whole grain flour cakes
- Whole couscous

WHOLE GRAIN CEREALS

- Whole grain oat flakes, wheat flakes, bran flakes, and so forth

*As described in chapter 2, white whole wheat flour is a whole grain flour with all of the nutritional benefits of traditional (red) whole wheat flour—not to be confused with refined, "white" all-purpose flour.

- Blends of whole grain cereals, either unsweetened or with whole sugar

NATURAL SWEETENERS

- Honey
- Whole sugar
- Maple syrup
- Blackstrap molasses
- Date syrup
- Pear concentrate
- Agave syrup
- Coconut sugar
- Malt (or barley) syrup
- Brown rice syrup
- Stevia

THE ORIGIN AND COMPOSITION OF SEVERAL NATURAL SWEETENERS

We should recall that for a sweetener to be considered natural, it should consist of not only the sweet molecules of the food but also their combination with other nutrients (vitamins, minerals, trace elements, and so on) in the original food. This is the case for the following sweeteners that are the most common. This is, however, far from an exhaustive list.

The sweeteners presented here are all natural, but that does not mean you can overindulge in them. They are very concentrated. By consuming them too often and too generously, you will not learn how to get rid of your sweet tooth.

Maple Syrup

Originating in the northeastern United States and Canada, maple syrup is made by boiling the sap of the sugar maple (*Acer saccharum*) to evaporate the water. It generally takes 40 gallons of sap to make 1 gallon of syrup (depending on the sugar content of the sap). The syrup consists of 69 percent carbohydrates, 68 percent of which is sucrose, 0.4 percent glucose, and 0.3 percent fructose. Maple syrup is rich in minerals and antioxidants, such as riboflavin, zinc, magnesium, calcium, manganese, thiamin, copper, and potassium.

Blackstrap Molasses

This is a thick liquid with a very syrupy consistency and a dark color that comes from the sap of sugarcane. It consists of 39 percent sucrose, 11 percent fructose, and 9 percent glucose. It contains a high quantity of minerals (9 percent of its weight) and vitamins. Blackstrap molasses is sold as a liquid or in the form of flakes or powder, and it has a very strong flavor.

Date Syrup

Date syrup is obtained by cooking dates with water, then by evaporating this fluid until it has boiled down to a thick syrup. This syrup consists of 39.6 percent glucose, 33.6 percent fructose, and 1.25 percent sucrose, as well as vitamins and minerals. It has a pleasant taste of dates.

Pear Concentrate

This sweetener is made in Switzerland with pear juice that has been reduced over heat into a syrup that has the consistency of liquid honey. It is 79 percent sugar, which consists of 70 percent sucrose, 7 percent fructose, and 2 percent glucose. It also contains vitamins and minerals. It retains the pleasant flavor of pears.

Agave Syrup

This syrup is produced from a cactus native to Mexico (*Agave tequilana*). Its sap is boiled down to the consistency of a thick syrup that is 56 percent fructose and 20 percent glucose. It also contains some vitamins and minerals. Its flavor is neutral.

Coconut Sugar

Native to Asia, this sugar is extracted from the nectar of coconut palm flowers. It consists of 75 percent sucrose, but also contains a little glucose (4 percent) and fructose (4 percent). It is rich in minerals. It is sold in the form of a powder with a caramel flavor.

Barley Malt Syrup

Malt syrup is manufactured from sprouted barley seeds that are dried and ground into a flour, which is then left to ferment. The starch of the flour transforms into sugar at this time, primarily maltose (65 percent). Maltose has the property of predigesting the starch of cereal grains and encouraging the production of milk in nursing women. The other sugars present are glucose (11 percent) and fructose (3 percent). Barley malt syrup also contains vitamins and minerals. It comes in the form of a sugary treacle that has the flavor of malt.

Brown Rice Syrup

This syrup is obtained from the fermentation of brown rice and barley. It comes in the form of a thick brown syrup that is 45 percent maltose and 3 percent glucose. It is very rich in vitamins and minerals and has a slight caramel flavor.

Stevia

Stevia is manufactured from the leaves of a plant (*Stevia rebaudiana*) that grows in Paraguay, and comes in the form of a powder or liquid. Stevia's sweetening power is not provided by its carbohydrates but by virtue of the plant's steviol glycosides, a substance that has enormous sweetening potential. This potential is 250 times stronger than that of sucrose (refined sugar). On the downside, some of the processing methods use chloroform, hydrochloric acid, or hexane (a crude-oil based solvent), and these are not required to be listed on the label.

Because it does not introduce any sugar into the body, it has no influence at all on blood sugar levels. It does not provide energy like other sugars, but is only used for its flavor to sweeten foods and beverages. It contains vitamins and minerals.

REPLACING BAD SUGARS WITH GOOD SUGARS

The replacement of bad sugars by good ones leads to the introduction of new consistencies or textures, as well as new flavors, all of which may take an adjustment period. Some people can have a hard time making the leap. The taste of these foods is not really enjoyable to them and they complain that they are either too strong, too bland, or just too different. Cooked foods seem too soft or too firm, and the cooking times are different.

In practice, though, when people make the effort to eat these foods regularly for several weeks, most of them end up liking most of the foods. Not only do they find them tasty, but they will often find that these foods with healthy sugars are better than the foods they ate before. This will become especially noticeable when they again eat a food that was once a regular part of their everyday diet. They will no longer enjoy the way it tastes. For example, yogurt with added sugar will taste too sweet, pasta made from refined white flour has no flavor, cookies taste like straight sugar and lack any flavor of the grains they are made from, and so forth.

This change in the way people perceive flavor will be long lasting. It will not fade over the passage of time but will grow stronger. And this is entirely normal, as the foods with good sugars are the very foods designed for our bodies by nature.

However, we must also take into consideration that we all have individual tastes. While all fruits are good for us, we will like some more than others. This holds true for all foods.

To facilitate the transition, there are a few pitfalls to avoid. For example, someone who has never eaten whole grain rice starts eating it, doesn't like it, and concludes that whole rice doesn't taste pleasing. However, there are many varieties of whole grain rice, with different flavors, textures, and consistencies. This individual has unfortunately started by eating a kind of whole grain rice that does not appeal, but that's not a good reason to abandon whole grain rice altogether. Among the many available, surely one or two will suit this person's taste buds.

Likewise, some people say they do not like whole grain rice because it is too hard. In fact, the problem is not that whole grain rice is naturally too hard—it is not—but that it has not been sufficiently cooked. The cooking process for whole grain rice is somewhat different from that of white rice. When its cooking time and heat have been adapted to meet its characteristics, whole grain rice has a pleasant consistency, as does any other kind of rice.

Whole grain pastas are made from different kinds of wheat, and can be prepared al dente or soft, according to taste. Here, too, it is necessary to test different kinds in order to find those with the most satisfying flavor and consistency.

The following table offers various possibilities for replacing bad sugars with good ones.

REPLACEMENT CHART

BAD SUGARS	GOOD SUGARS
Refined sugars: white, brown	Whole sugars: honey, maple syrup, blackstrap molasses, and so on
Artificial sweeteners	Stevia
Refined cereal grains	Whole grain cereals
All-purpose flour and blends	Whole wheat flour, whole rye flour, and so on
White and mostly white bread	Whole grain and mostly whole grain bread
White flour crackers, Saltines, water crackers	Whole grain crackers
White pasta	Whole grain pasta
White cake flour	Whole grain cake flour
Breakfast cereal with refined sugar	Breakfast flakes without sugar or with whole sugar or honey
Cake made with refined sugar	Whole grain cake with dried fruits; sweetened with honey, whole sugar, or barley malt syrup
Cookies made with refined sugar	Whole grain cookies with dried fruit and nuts
Pastries	Whole grain pastries sweetened with honey, whole sugar, or barley malt syrup
Ice cream	Homemade ice cream sweetened with honey, whole sugar, or fruit; yogurt or cottage cheese with whole sugar, honey, and so on
Sweetened chocolate bar	Fresh or dried fruits, whole grain cookies with whole sugar, dark chocolate bars (>80 percent cacao)
Candies	Fresh fruits, dried fruits, mixed dried fruits

BAD SUGARS	GOOD SUGARS
Nutella	Pure almond, cashew, or hazelnut butter
Commercial tomato puree, ketchup, barbecue sauce	Ketchup and sauces with no added sugar
Fruit juice with added sugar	Pure, natural fruit juices
Commercial soft drinks, iced teas, sport beverages	Homemade herb or black teas sweetened with honey or whole sugar, pure fruit juices with sparkling water, or unsweetened fruit-flavored sparkling water
Coffee, tea, herb tea with sugar	Coffee, tea, herb tea without sugar or with whole sugar or honey

Replacing bad sugars with good sugars is not only beneficial for your health, it also allows you to discover new foods and new flavors.

11

EATING ENOUGH SLOW SUGARS

Goal: To eat enough slow sugars to provide your body with the energy it needs over the long term.

The notion of fast sugars and slow sugars has been challenged with the creation of the glycemic index (GI) system. This is why I will first present in this chapter the traditional way of introducing them, then tackle the issues that have arisen from the glycemic index approach.

FAST AND SLOW SUGARS, TRADITIONAL NOTIONS

Foods that are high in carbohydrates provide the body with the energy it needs. They are its fuel and there are two kinds of fuel: light and heavy.

The light fuel consists of foods that are rich in monosaccharides and disaccharides, which is to say glucose, fructose, and sucrose. These foods are fruits, sweet vegetables (carrots and so forth), and milk. The very simple chemical structure of these molecules makes it so they have practically no need of being digested. They are either directly available as is or require only minor transformation. They therefore can rapidly travel through the mucous membranes of the intestines to enter the bloodstream. The speed with which these sugars become physiologically available has earned them the name of "fast sugars."

The heavy fuel comes from foods that are high in starch, made from the combination of large numbers of glucose molecules (up to 250,000 units). We find starch in grains, leguminous foods, potatoes, chestnuts, and so forth. Starch has a very elaborate structure with long chains that must be cut into smaller and smaller segments until they are broken down to isolated molecules of glucose that the bloodstream is able to absorb. Because the glucose can become available only gradually from this source, it is called "slow sugar."

Fast sugars are a light fuel, not only because they are quickly absorbed but also because they are quickly burned away. Someone who eats only apples to get energy will only receive glucose for a short interval of time. The body will quickly burn it, which contributes nothing to maintaining an optimum blood sugar level. This individual will very soon be again in need of sugar and energy. A light fuel only supplies energy for the short term. This is not the kind of fuel that must be eaten to maintain sufficient energy to get through a whole day.

Things are different for the slow sugars. They are digested slowly. The glucose enters the bloodstream gradually over a period of hours. This slow rhythm ensures that the bloodstream receives glucose over a long period to maintain a steady blood sugar level. The individual is receiving energy continuously, thus there is no need to eat again right away to obtain sugar. Slow sugars are therefore clearly the "heavy fuel" that we need for the long term.

A good illustration of this can be seen among bicycle racers. Before competitions they eat large quantities of pasta (called "carb loading")—not apples—to support the enormous physical efforts they will have to make. We also see this among manual laborers, who are big eaters of grains, potatoes, beans, bread, and proteins rather than fruits and vegetables that provide only a light fuel.

To ensure having enough energy at your disposal for the whole day, it is therefore necessary to eat slow sugars on a regular basis. Eating these slow sugars is particularly recommended at breakfast, as this will permit you to have enough energy for the entire morning.

Some people totally refuse to do this, however. They mistakenly believe that foods with slow sugars (grains, potatoes) have all sorts of drawbacks: that they cause weight gain, are full of toxins, and so forth. Or even that the gluten in grains is harmful for everyone when it is only the case for those who are allergic to it. Having made the decision to not eat slow sugars, or very little of them, these people fall back almost exclusively on fast sugars. However, these sugars do not give them enough energy and they must be constantly ingesting them, with the danger, if they are bad sugars (sweets, chocolates), of becoming intoxicated and suffering from attacks of reactive hypoglycemia.

FAST AND SLOW SUGARS ACCORDING TO THE GLYCEMIC INDEX APPROACH

The measures that are taken to determine the glycemic index ranking of foods have provided some surprising results. Curiously, they seem to have called into question the validity of the very notion of fast and slow sugars.

Fruits, which until this index was established had been considered fast sugars, were given a low GI ranking. This low GI is supposed to mean that the sugars enter the bloodstream slowly because the blood sugar level scarcely rises. For this reason they would seem to be slow sugars, not fast sugars.

Conversely, potatoes and rice, which were earlier considered to be slow sugars, have a high GI ranking. In other words, the glucose released by these foods is considered to be rapidly available and tangibly raise blood sugar levels. This would suggest they are not slow sugars but fast sugars.

At first glance, this would seem to provide positive proof that the notion of fast sugars and slow sugars was demonstrably false, as they act in a way that is opposite to what their names indicate. But in reality this is not the case. The glycemic index system only provides indications of a food's ability to raise blood sugar level, but none concerning the time with which it takes to deliver its glucose. It only takes one factor of the equation into account, whereas in reality there are two. This second factor is fundamental. In fact, if it is recommended that athletes eat slow sugars, it is because that will provide them energy over a long period of time. This is precisely what happens with slow sugars, independent of the food's glycemic index.

The GI of potatoes, for example, gives the impression of fast sugars, as the glucose they provide quickly enters the bloodstream (hence their elevated GI). But the timeframe during which potatoes provide glucose to the body is a long one. Because the body uses this glucose slowly, it is therefore a slow sugar.

The low GI of apples indicates that they are a slow sugar. In fact, the blood sugar level rise they cause is slight because the sugar enters the bloodstream quite slowly. But while they do enter the bloodstream slowly, the time during which they do so is very *short*. The glucose provided by an apple is quickly used up; hence it is a fast sugar.

In the traditional approach, the terms *fast* and *slow* are primarily used to define the speed with which the sugar is used by the body; in the glycemic index system, the terms refer to the speed with which the glucose enters the bloodstream.

The notion of fast and slow sugars should consequently not

be considered to be wrong. They are still perfectly appropriate and of great practical use when you are looking for foods that will give you energy over the long term.

LIST OF FOODS WITH SLOW SUGARS

- Whole wheat
- Whole rye
- Whole oats
- Whole barley
- Whole corn
- Whole rice
- Whole spelt
- Whole millet
- Whole buckwheat
- Whole quinoa
- Whole grain bread
- Whole grain crackers
- Cereal flakes
- Whole grain pastas
- Potatoes
- Chestnuts
- Soybeans
- Lentils

The body needs equal amounts of both fast and slow sugars to fill its energy needs, but also because eating a varied diet allows us to benefit from a much larger range of nutrients.

12

ADDING PROTEINS TO EXTEND THE GLYCEMIC CURVE

Goal: To maintain a heightened energy level over a long period of time by adding proteins to the carbohydrates you eat for breakfast.

Everyone likes having enough energy for performing daily tasks. We also are living in a fast-paced society that demands everyone be in top form, which also requires having enough energy.

Many people, however, do not have all the energy they want or need at their disposal. They are easily wearied and lack vitality and strength. Empty stretches and sudden onsets of fatigue appear regularly during their days. They lack tone and exhaust themselves quickly. Their glycemic curve barely manages to stay at a horizontal level over the course of the day. It slumps too quickly and often threatens to fall into the zone of hypoglycemia.

What can these people do to have more energy and, what's more, energy that lasts for a considerably longer period of time?

The level of strength we have available over the course of the day depends on what kind of fuel we are giving our bodies—in other words, what kinds of foods we are eating. This is why countless studies have been performed to analyze the effect of different kinds of meals, and more specifically breakfast, on blood sugar levels.

THE EFFECT OF BREAKFAST ON BLOOD SUGAR LEVEL

In a 1949 study by E. Orent-Keiles and L. F. Hallman published by the U.S. Department of Agriculture, around two hundred volunteers were divided into groups. Each group was served a different breakfast. The blood sugar level of the study participants was measured before the meal (thus on an empty stomach), then once an hour for three hours following breakfast.

The members of the first group broke their fast with nothing but black coffee. Their blood sugar level on an empty stomach was not very high to begin with and spiked briefly before falling continuously over the course of the morning. The majority of the volunteers in this group felt lethargic and lacked strength.

The members of the second group were given a menu corresponding to what might be considered a typical American breakfast: orange juice, toast with butter and jelly, two small slices of bacon, and coffee with cream and sugar. Initially their blood sugar level rose quickly, but after around an hour it began to decline. For many of the participants of this group, it fell back to a level below that of the blood sugar level they had on an empty stomach, and it remained there for the rest of the morning. The members of this group had no energy and were ineffective all morning.

A third group received the same menu as the second group but with the addition of oatmeal with milk and sugar. Here again, the blood sugar level spiked rapidly but quickly fell below that of the other group. The lack of energy that resulted persisted throughout the entire morning as well.

In the fourth group, the members were served the earlier described American-style breakfast but accompanied by two eggs. The blood sugar rose and stabilized at 1.20 grams (normal being 0.8 grams to 1.1 grams)—in other words, a good level—which allowed the participants of this group to enjoy sufficient energy and a sense of well-being until the middle of the day.

For the fifth group, the eggs were replaced by two tablespoons of milk enriched with powdered milk. Their blood sugar levels also rose to 1.20 grams and remained there the entire morning.

These experiments show that the exclusive consumption of carbohydrates at breakfast is not the most efficient way of gaining and maintaining energy. The blood sugar level climbs, even rapidly, but it is not able to maintain itself at this level to provide energy over the long term. Conversely, adding proteins to the carbohydrates stabilizes the blood sugar level and makes it possible to enjoy a good deal of energy over a long period of time.

The practical conclusion that can be drawn from these experiments is that the carbohydrates of the breakfast meal should be topped off by a source of protein for best results in maintaining sufficient energy levels over the course of the morning.

PROTEINS AND CARBOHYDRATES

Why do proteins have such a beneficial influence on blood sugar levels?

Carbohydrate foods, protein foods, and lipid foods all require different digestive juices to be digested properly. When several of these juices are present in the intestinal tract at the same time, they can impede each other. The digestive processes can be slowed almost to a standstill. The foods are digested more slowly and consequently are slower to enter the bloodstream. On the other hand, when the foods eaten all belong to the same type, the digestive juices act without any hindrance. The nutrients are quickly digested and made available to the body, facilitating more rapid passage into the bloodstream.

This is why a breakfast consisting only of carbohydrate foods can be digested in a short while, especially if these foods also contain bad sugars. A great deal of sugar is made physiologically available very quickly and enters the bloodstream. This forces the pancreas to react strongly, which has the result of lowering the blood sugar level.

In contrast, when the breakfast consists of both carbohydrates and proteins, the action of the digestive juices responsible for digestion of the carbohydrates is hindered by those that are acting on the proteins. The glucose released from the digestion process is made available gradually, so it enters the bloodstream slowly and in small quantities. The blood sugar level therefore rises gradually and remains at a good level.

Two reasons explain the stability of the blood sugar level that results from mixing carbohydrates with proteins. On the one hand, the glucose is released only gradually from the alimentary bolus because of the decelerated rate of the digestive process. The foods therefore make their way to the bloodstream little by little over a long period of time. There they replace what has already been used up, which helps maintain the blood sugar level. On the other hand, the slow and measured entry of glucose into the bloodstream does not prompt the pancreas to overreact. The release of insulin is normal and does not create a drop in the blood sugar level.

Proteins therefore have a regulating effect on the use of sugars by lengthening the glycemic curve. Rather than sharply falling shortly after breakfast, as is often the case when only carbohydrates are consumed, the blood sugar level remains the same for a considerable period of time.

Thanks to the regulatory effect of proteins, it's clearly unnecessary to eat huge amounts of carbohydrates in order to get energy. It is enough to consume what is a normal quantity for you, but combined with proteins.

Some people will be surprised to read that exclusive consumption of carbohydrates at breakfast will bring about a drop in the blood sugar level around an hour later. They say they have never seen that reaction in themselves. There are two possible explanations for this. The first is that these individuals are eating whole carbohydrates, therefore slow sugars, which is to say good sugars, contrary to what was the case during the experiments cited earlier. The pancreas did not overreact and there was no sudden drop in the blood sugar level caused by an excessive release of insulin.

The second reason is that many people eat a snack midmorning, before the effects of hypoglycemia make themselves fully felt. In this case the snack causes the blood sugar level to rise.

THE REGULATING ROLE OF PROTEINS

The fundamental influence of proteins is not solely on hypoglycemia, but on quite a few different processes.

It has been observed among diabetics with insufficient consumption of proteins that raising the protein intake helped them to metabolize carbohydrates much more effectively, resulting in a reduction of the quantity of sugar that collected in their bloodstream. Here the regulatory role of the proteins went to work against hyperglycemia, and not on hypoglycemia.

Some people lose minerals easily because they have trouble neutralizing the weak acids of fruits, yogurt, and vinegar. In its efforts to neutralize these acids the body expends a large amount of its alkaline substances, which causes the loss of minerals. Empirical evidence shows, however, that this tendency to become acidic and lose minerals is greater when the individual consumes very little protein. The evidence also shows that increasing protein intake makes their bodies much more able to neutralize the weak acids.

Proteins also have a role in the digestive organs. Quantitative and qualitative fine-tuning of protein intake often succeeds in curing someone who has been suffering from chronic indigestion, even when the changes mandated by a large variety of other diets has utterly failed and protein regulating is undertaken as a last resort.

FOODS WITH PROTEIN

There are many foods that are high in proteins, and they come in all flavors. Some are of animal origin and others come from plants. Generally speaking, the first are more beneficial against hypoglycemia than the second. The reason is that proteins from animal sources have the nine essential amino acids, which is not generally the case with those from plant sources. The proteins animal sources offer are better used and therefore the protein intake is greater.

The choice of protein foods is very personal. They are chosen in accordance with taste as well as, for some, ethical preference, but also for one's ability to eat them for breakfast. While some people can eat bacon or sausages early in the morning without any problem, others cannot and are satisfied with eggs or cheese. That said, processed meats such as bacon and sausage are not the most highly recommended foods for maintaining good health, no matter when they are eaten!

PROTEIN FOODS AND
THEIR PROTEIN CONTENT

FOOD	PERCENTAGE OF PROTEINS
Beans	20–33%
Cheese	20–30%
Meat	18–22%
Oleaginous foods	14–18%
Fish	13–20%
Grains	8–14%
Yogurt	10%
Eggs	6–7%
Milk	3.4%

Different Ways to Eat Protein in the Morning

Foods high in proteins can be eaten in a multitude of ways. The chart below provides a number of different options for each kind of food. Proteins allow breakfast to be a savory meal.

Milk (for children*)	Plain, or blended with fruit as a smoothie
Yogurt	Plain, with fresh or dried fruits, nuts, seeds, granola
Cheese	Cottage cheese: with fresh or dried fruits, nuts, seeds, cereal flakes, herbs, vegetables Spreadable cheese, cream cheese: on bread or crackers Hard or soft cheese: with bread or crackers
Meat	Sliced fresh ham, chicken
Fish	Herring, tuna, salmon
Egg	Poached, soft- or hard-boiled, fried, scrambled, in an omelet

*Adults cannot digest milk correctly; the enzyme necessary for proper digestion of milk stops being produced by the stomach between seven and ten years of age.

13

MAKING BREAKFAST A PRIORITY

Goal: To make yourself a good breakfast so you can have a high energy level all day long.

Of the three meals of the day, breakfast should be the priority. While it is perfectly true that mixing proteins with carbohydrates is beneficial for blood sugar levels at any meal, it is particularly good at breakfast. A variety of experiments have clearly shown that our energy level over the course of the day depends heavily on what kinds of foods we eat for breakfast.

A REVEALING EXPERIMENT

The experiments described in the preceding chapter were designed to determine the effect of different breakfasts on blood sugar levels during the period that directly followed the meal—in other words, over the course of the morning. An additional experiment was conducted by the same researchers to discover what kind of impact breakfast might have on the rest of the day. To determine this, the same volunteers were given an identical meal at noon and thereafter their blood sugar level readings were taken every hour. The meal consisted of whole grain bread for the carbohydrate portion, with cottage cheese and a glass of milk for protein.

Because the same meal was provided for all the volunteers, it could be expected that its effect on blood sugar levels would be the same for everyone over the course of the afternoon, but this was not the case. Of course, everyone experienced the same immediate effect: the blood sugar level rose slightly directly following the meal. However, a short time later, the blood sugar level behaved differently, according to the kind of breakfast the volunteer had eaten.

The volunteers whose breakfast had caused their blood sugar levels to climb to a good point and remain there all morning (groups 4 and 5) saw their good blood sugar levels extended for the entire afternoon. They therefore had plenty of energy at their disposal. This is termed the second-meal phenomenon.

On the other hand, for a large number of the participants (groups 1, 2, and 3), whose blood sugar level had soon dropped following the exclusive consumption of carbohydrates, after the spike in the blood level caused by lunch, the sugar content diminished back to the same levels as experienced in the morning. In other words, their blood sugar levels remained low all day, and they felt weak and lethargic until the evening.

The conclusion drawn by this experiment has great practical value: a breakfast consisting of both protein and carbohydrates not only ensures a good energy level during the morning but also is conducive to keeping energy levels consistently high during the afternoon.

A breakfast that mixes carbohydrates and proteins is therefore preferable, energetically speaking, to a breakfast that consists solely of carbohydrates. The importance of breakfast in comparison to the other meals of the day clearly bears out the old maxim that advises people to eat breakfast like a king, lunch like a prince, and dinner like a pauper.

A WORLD TOUR
OF AN AMPLE BREAKFAST

Human beings did not wait for the experiments just described to realize the benefits of mixing carbohydrates with proteins. Many peoples, all across the globe, have made this discovery through their own experience and created their own kinds of morning meal as a result. Note that in the following examples the carbohydrates consumed include both fast sugars and slow sugars (see chapter 11) that encourage energy production over the long term.

The English and Americans eat bacon and eggs as well as toast with butter and jelly. In Germany and Austria, slices of bread with jam are accompanied by cold cuts and cheese. In the Scandinavian countries, people eat bread with fish, cheese, or meat. In Brazil, we again find bread, butter, and jelly with cheese and cold cuts. In the Philippines, breakfast consists of mangos, rice, and sausages, which are accompanied by a pancake made from rice, eggs, meat, and beans. In Morocco, people eat different kinds of bread with jam and cheese. In China, rice or noodles sautéed with chicken and vegetables is a common morning entry. In Uganda we find bananas cooked with beef and vegetables. A traditional Japanese breakfast includes grilled fish, rice, and seaweed.

It is also interesting to look at what is eaten by people who use a lot of physical energy during the day. For example, many manual laborers at their 9:00 a.m. break eat bread, sausage, and cheese, a meal that has both carbohydrates and proteins to provide them with enough energy to perform their demanding work.

LACK OF APPETITE IN THE MORNING

Some people will object that while they would really like to eat a good breakfast combining proteins and carbohydrates, unfortunately they have no appetite so early in the day.

Often these are the same people who are content with simply drinking a coffee to start the day off "right." But as we saw earlier, having nothing but coffee for breakfast is not beneficial. In the beginning there is clearly a rise of the blood sugar level as coffee stimulates the conversion of glycogen into glucose by acting on the adrenal glands. However, the rapid entry of the glucose into the bloodstream compels a strong reaction from the pancreas. The large quantity of insulin it releases then causes the blood sugar level of most people to tumble precipitously, taking their energy level along with it. Drinking another cup of coffee as a pick-me-up will again only be effective for the short term.

Other people have no appetite in the morning but do not turn to coffee to begin their day. They satisfy themselves with eating "a little something" that is so small it has no influence on the blood sugar level and consequently does not prompt the pancreas to react. The people in this case can enjoy a completely satisfying energy level because their bodies are in the habit of converting glycogen into glucose all morning long in order to maintain an optimum blood sugar level.

But this encompasses only a small minority of people. Others really need breakfast to be in shape until noon. But what about those who are not hungry in the morning? What should they do?

The primary reason for the lack of appetite in the morning is often that the evening meal is too plentiful. Not only is it too plentiful, it is also eaten too late in the evening. The digestive process therefore starts late and continues over a large part of the night. In some cases it is only completed just as the person is waking up for the following day. In these conditions it is normal that the people concerned would have no appetite and not be hungry. Contrary to what would be good for them, these people have a dinner fit for a king and not a pauper, and a breakfast fit for a pauper, not a king.

To reverse matters it is necessary to eat less and not so late at night. Initially someone making this change may perhaps suffer a little from not eating as big a dinner as before, but this is primarily a question of habit. The individual may have the impression of not getting enough nourishment, which is good, in fact, because in the morning there will be a feeling of hunger. The appetite these individuals feel then will ensure that they eat a good breakfast. Over time, meal habits will change and breakfast will take a more important place and dinner less.

For other people the problem is not eating too much at dinner, but they snack all evening in front of the television. Here, too, a change is necessary; they must abstain from snacking the night before in order to have an appetite in the morning.

There is another category of people, however, who, no matter what they do, have no appetite in the morning. These are people whose bodies have difficulty resuming their normal functioning rhythm after resting all night. They have trouble getting up out of bed. They are still functioning in slow motion. A certain amount of time is necessary for these people to recover their normal rhythm.

This physiological weakness of the morning is not inevitable or inescapable. It can be corrected. The body has great powers of adaptability and a person can become accustomed to becoming functional more quickly in the morning. It is worth the trouble to take the necessary steps to adjust this way, as a good breakfast is essential, for most people, to having enough energy in the morning.

The way to proceed for these people is to force themselves to eat something, even if in the beginning it is simply a little snack: a cracker, some almonds, a little cottage cheese, or yogurt. This demand forces the body to respond. Over time it will become used to it and breakfast can gradually become larger. It will certainly never be as abundant as the breakfast of a hearty eater, but eventually it will come to resemble a normal breakfast. To reach this goal you must stick with it for several weeks, but the benefit that results is more energy and greater zest for life. This is truly worth the trouble.

14

EVALUATING OTHER CAUSES OF ENERGY DEPLETION AND SUGAR CRAVINGS

Goal: To discover other reasons that could be the cause of your low energy—and how to fix it.

Hypoglycemia is not the only reason we lack energy and are driven to eat sweet foods in order to recover our strength.

There can be other reasons:

- dehydration
- an acid-alkaline imbalance
- a sedentary lifestyle

When we feel lethargic, we naturally seek to address the situation. Unfortunately we are not always aware of the true causes for this fatigue. We think maybe it's caused by low blood sugar so we eat sugar, but the lack of sugar is not necessarily responsible for our lack of energy. Also, the sugars we choose for this energy boost are, generally speaking, bad sugars, which only increases overconsumption of carbohydrates with no benefit.

People who often feel fatigued and without energy need to try to determine if one or more of the factors described in this chapter are at work in their situation. They will then be able to take steps to address these factors, and thereby reduce their sugar consumption.

DEHYDRATION

Our bodies consist of 70 percent water. To function properly, they must regularly take in more water to replace the fluid that is eliminated via urine, stools, perspiration, and breathing. For most people the intake is not sufficient to keep up with these eliminations. These people do not drink enough and they become dehydrated. Energy loss is one of the metabolic disorders that is created by poor hydration. This loss of vigor is due to the fact that the enzymes can no longer work properly.

Enzymes are responsible for all the biochemical transformations that take place in the body. They act as catalysts; that is, they speed up biochemical reactions. They are therefore indispensable in the processes of digestion, absorption, cellular multiplication, defense, and so forth, as well as for the production of energy. To properly perform their work, enzymes require an environment that has high water content. This gives them sufficient space to activate and perform their work effectively.

Conversely, the more their working space is reduced due to a lack of fluid, the greater difficulty enzymes have in successfully completing their tasks, as the bodily fluids are too thick and congested. This heightened viscosity is the inevitable result of dehydration.

When enzymes find themselves in a restrictive environment that hampers their activity, they continue to work, but at a slower pace. Over time this rhythm slows down and the biochemical transformations are performed imperfectly and intermittently. In the worst-case scenario, they stop completely.

This enzymatic slowdown can paralyze the entire organic processes of the body, as all the activities necessary for its proper functioning, including—and this is what is important for our subject—the production of energy, gradually diminish. In this way the lack of sufficient water in the body leads to a lack of energy.

This energy deficit manifests as fatigue, lack of enthusiasm, the desire to do nothing, and the impression of not being up to performing your daily duties. The mental state is also altered, manifesting as a lack of passion and joy in life and work.

The influence of dehydration on physical capabilities has been calculated very precisely in sports medicine. The figures resulting from these studies clearly demonstrate how quickly dehydration has an adverse influence on physiological function. All the body needs is a fluid loss equivalent to 1 percent of body weight for abilities to decline by 10 percent. When there is a loss of 2 percent of body weight, effectiveness declines by 20 percent. This weakening continues at the same rhythm until around 10 percent of body weight, the stage at which the dehydrated individual loses consciousness and all physical and motor capabilities. Beyond this threshold physiological disorders accelerate and lead to death.

? Did You Know?

For a person weighing 155 pounds, 1 percent of body weight represents only 0.7 quarts of water, a quantity of fluid that is easily lost through sweat during an hour of physical exercise at an ambient temperature of around 64°F. At 82°F the hydric loss will border on three quarts an hour; in other words, 4 percent of body weight and a 40 percent loss of physical capacity. Someone who is a chronic sufferer of dehydration is therefore constantly suffering from lack of energy.

REDUCTION OF THE ABILITY TO WORK
BASED ON THE LOSS OF WATER

**ABILITY TO WORK
IN RELATION TO THE NORM
(IN PERCENT)**

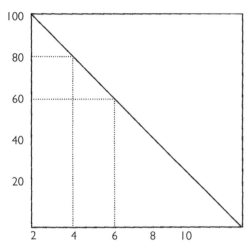

LOSS OF FLUID (IN PERCENT OF BODY WEIGHT)

Source: L. Hermanse, cited in Alan Garnier, *Alimentation et Sport*

In the case of dehydration, the cause of the energy deficit being the lack of water, the obvious solution would be to increase the intake of water. This is really the only effective solution, because it addresses the very root of the problem. In fact, it is only by removing the cause that the effects are alleviated.

In other words, someone suffering from low energy can rehydrate by drinking enough liquid every day and recover all former strength. A generous intake of water (2.5 quarts a day) will in fact relaunch enzymatic activity and allow a heightened level of energy to return. A resurgence of strength and vitality is one of the first effects mentioned by most people who have increased their water consumption to bring hydration levels back to normal.

However, many people will not take this step. They do not heed the sensation of thirst their body gives them to let them know it needs more fluids and that it is imperative to get them. To the contrary, these people often confuse thirst and hunger and eat—bad sugars in particular—instead of drinking water. This provides temporary relief, but not because of the carbohydrates they have ingested, as they were not responsible for their lack of energy. These people recovered their strength for other reasons. On the one hand, it is because almost all foods contain water, something the body was lacking at that time. On the other, it is because the pancreas and the body went into a state of alert when confronted by the arrival of bad sugars, which stimulated the body and gave it a temporary burst of energy.

The consumption of these sugars can therefore be easily avoided if people drink something when feeling low in energy, rather than eat. If they take this step, they will see that their fatigue actually vanishes.*

> People who are fatigued because they are dehydrated should drink water rather than eat sugar to restore their energy levels.

THE LOSS OF THE ACID-ALKALINE BALANCE

An acid-alkaline imbalance in the body is another cause of lack of energy and a craving to eat sweets.

The substances that compose the human body are either acidic or alkaline. The body will not function properly unless both these types of substances are present in equal

---

*For more on this, see my book *The Water Prescription* (Healing Arts Press, 2006).

quantities, hence the notion of the acid-alkaline balance.

In our era of overeating, sedentary lifestyles, stress, and so forth, this balance is prone to being disrupted by an increase of acidic substances. It is extremely rare for the opposite situation to occur, which would mean this balance is threatened by alkalosis (too much alkaline). When this does happen, the cause is generally a serious disease.

A greater variety of organic functional disorders can result from the acidification of the body's cellular terrain (acidosis). This first crops up as minor health problems: dry skin, hair loss, brittle nails, nervousness, and so on. But over time and increased acidification, health disorders will become more severe: tendinitis, neuritis, rheumatism, depressive states, and, most importantly, fatigue and a loss of energy.

The lack of energy and lethargy, tiring easily and recovering slowly, are typical symptoms of an acidified terrain. This fatigue appears in the same way as that resulting from intense physical effort. The repeated contractions of the muscles produce lactic acid. The presence of this acid causes the muscles to tire. This is a means of protection used by nature to avoid too much wear and tear on the muscles in too short a time by obliging us to rest. This phenomenon is valid for the entire body; a body suffering from acidosis is an exhausted body. It is fatigued not because it has used up too much energy but because it is acidic.

Here again, the cause of this energy deficit results from the reduction of energy production by the enzymes.

There is an ideal pH for the body, and more specifically for its cellular terrain, that allows the enzymes to function at an optimum level. (The pH measures the degree of a substance's acidity or alkalinity.) Any change of the pH will inevitably lead to an alteration in enzymatic activity, which most often is expressed by it slowing down. The more acidic the terrain becomes, the more the enzymes are hindered and shackled. Among other things, they are then less capable of producing energy.

This is why a person suffering from slight acidification feels tired, but someone who is seriously acidified is experiencing a true loss of energy. Both individuals naturally look for a way to restore their strength. If they are not aware of the true cause of their fatigue—acidity—they will eat, thinking that they have run out of fuel. The foods they choose are likely to be high in sugar, and unfortunately, for most people these will be bad sugars.

In this vicious cycle a person suffering from acidification is eating bad sugars when the lack of sugar is not the cause of their lack of energy. This consumption makes things worse in the long term because the bad sugars make the terrain more acidic.

The real solution then would be the elimination of the cause of their exhaustion by restoring a healthy acid-alkaline balance. In concrete terms, this means stopping the acids at their source by a change of diet and thus eliminating excess acids in the body.

The reformation of the diet is based on the reduction of acidifying foods (sweets, white bread, meat, fried foods) and increase of alkalizing foods (green and colored vegetables, potatoes, nuts, fruits).

The elimination of acids is obtained by stimulating the organs responsible for their elimination: the kidneys and the skin. This can be achieved through the use of diuretic plants and sessions of intense sweating (saunas and hot soaks). Finally, taking alkaline supplements will make it possible to effectively neutralize the acids lodged in the tissues.*

---

*For more on this, see my book *The Acid-Alkaline Diet for Optimum Health* (Healing Arts Press, 2006.)

By restoring the acid-alkaline balance using these various measures, your fatigue will disappear and your energy levels will bounce back to normal. Your craving for sugar will also vanish.

Individuals who are exhausted because they are acidified should focus on eliminating excess acids. They should resist eating sweet foods to recover their energy.

A SEDENTARY LIFESTYLE

As we go about our daily chores and expend energy, the glucose in the bloodstream is used by the cells, so it is inevitable that its level will drop. But the need for the cells to refuel doesn't stop. This is why, when blood sugar level reaches the normal bottom limit, which is to say 0.8 grams per liter, glucose must absolutely be provided to the bloodstream. This can be done either by intake of sugar via the consumption of sugar-rich foods or the body can extract these sugars from itself. In the latter case, it transforms the glycogen stored in the liver and muscles into glucose, which then enters the bloodstream.

The conversion of glycogen into glucose takes place whenever necessary during the course of the day, depending on level of exertion. The body particularly relies on this measure when engaged in intense physical activities. When this effort is pushed to extremes, as is often the case with athletes, the body must seek deeper within itself for stored sugar. The ability to convert glycogen into glucose improves every time the body does this, if only by a little. Eventually the active person's body will be clearly superior at performing this conversion process than the body of someone who rarely engages in physical activities.

> By engaging in a certain amount of physical activity, people who lead sedentary lives can teach their bodies how to draw sugar from their reserves.

Among people who lead a sedentary lifestyle, the opposite is what happens. As they never put any demand on their reserves, their ability to do so diminishes. Over time it becomes quite weak. The result of this phenomenon is a total or partial incapacity to draw from its reserves when blood sugar levels fall below their normal range. This accentuates the drop of blood sugar causing a craving for sugar to manifest, and the person affected starts eating something sweet. This consumption of sugars—which here, too, often consists of bad sugars—takes place even though the individual has no real need to eat them. In fact, the body's glycogen reserves are not empty. The problem is only that the body is unable to make use of these reserves because it has lost the habit. It struggles to do so—and does it poorly—only during intensive physical efforts, and very little if at all when no physical activity is prompting the body to release its reserves.

The best means for improving the body's ability to draw from its existing reserves is to get regular exercise. This could be a sport practiced outside in nature or simple physical exercises such as walking, gardening, or going on a bike ride. The repeated contractions of the muscles will burn away the sugar available in the bloodstream. You will start feeling sensations of fatigue and hunger, but if you resist and don't eat anything, but just continue exerting yourself, it will force the body to react. It will transform stored glycogen into glucose. At first this process will be minimal and poorly performed; then, with repetition, it will start releasing larger quantities over longer periods of time. Finally, once the body is accustomed again to performing this task, it will be able to do so even when there are no physical activities triggering it, simply when blood sugar levels start dropping a little too steeply. At this point, resorting to bad sugars between meals to restore the proper blood sugar level will no longer be necessary. The body will take charge of restoring the blood sugar content to a healthy level by dipping into its reserves.

CONCLUSION

The harmful effects of refined sugar are becoming more widely known every day. Not only have a growing number of individuals become aware of this, but it has become a source of concern to our governments.

Pressure has been applied to the manufacturers of foods that are high in refined sugar to lower its content in their products. In the United States, France, and an increasing number of other countries, products that are high in refined sugar or corn syrup, sodas for example, are being taxed. As is the case with alcohol and tobacco, the purpose of a high tax is to help persuade people to stop or reduce their use of these products. The goal is to reduce their consumption by raising their prices. Hopefully this will be more successful with sugar than it has been with tobacco, where soaring prices have decreased consumption only minimally.

These measures are beneficial, but they do not absolve people from the need to take responsibility for their own health. In the final analysis it is always up to the individual to either choose poor food options that result in illness or to eat sensibly and stay healthy by eliminating or reducing consumption of refined sugar and replacing it with the good sugars offered by nature.

We are fortunate to live in a country and a time that continues to present more and more options of tasty and nutritious foods in our markets, with many markets offering a salad bar and healthy prepared foods for days we're not inclined to cook. We've also got numerous restaurant and grocery home delivery services just a phone call away. And we've had explosive growth in farmers markets—76 percent increase in the national directory since 2008—offering fresh and inviting arrays of locally grown produce at reasonable prices. It may take a bit more effort initially, but with so many splendid options, we'd be foolish not to take advantage of them, and in so doing, take the best possible care of ourselves. What we eat today is truly our health tomorrow.

BIBLIOGRAPHY

Béguin, Dr. Max-Henri. *Mon enfant aura de bonnes dents.* La Chaux-de-Fonds, Switzerland: Édition de l'étoile, 1989.

Carton, Paul. *Traité de médicine, d'alimentation et d'hygiène naturistes.* Paris: Maloine, 1931.

Dufty, William. *Le sucre, cet ami qui vous veut du mal.* Paris: Éditions Trédaniel, 2006.

Garnier, Alan. *Alimentation et Sport.* Paris: Maloine, 1992.

Montignac, Michel. *La méthode Montignac.* Quebec: Flammarion, 2006.

Nittler, Alan H. *A New Breed of Doctor.* New York: Pyramid House, 1972.

Price, Weston A. *Nutrition and Physical Degeneration.* Lemon Grove, Calif.: Price Pottenger, 2008.

Starenkyj, Danièle. *Le mal du sucre.* Québec: Orion Publications, 1999.

Vasey, Christopher. *The Water Prescription.* Rochester, Vt.: Healing Arts Press, 2006.

———. *The Acid-Alkaline Diet for Optimum Health.* Rochester, Vt.: Healing Arts Press, 2006.

Yudkin, John. *Pure, White, and Deadly.* New York: Penguin, 2012.

INDEX

Page numbers in *italics* indicate illustrations, tables, or charts.

acid-alkaline balance
  loss of, and energy, 154–57
  maintaining, 60–62, *61*
acidosis, 68–69
addiction and refined sugar, 83–86
adrenal glands and regulation of
  blood sugar, 55, *55,* 56, 76, 147
agave syrup, *94,* 125, 127
alcohol dependency, 83–86
alkaline balance. *See* acid-alkaline
  balance
allergies. *See also* gluten sensitivity
  acids and, 62
  to nuts, coconut flour for, 37
Americas, sugarcane plantations
  in, 13–14
animal starch, 43
appetite
  intense, 68
  lack of, 146–49
artificial sweeteners. *See* sweeteners
aspartame. *See* sweeteners

barley malt syrup. *See* maltose
  (malt sugar)
basmati rice, *95,* 101. *See also*
  brown rice
beets, sugar. *See* sugar beets
beverages with refined sugar, 111
blackstrap molasses. *See* molasses
blood pressure
  acids and, 62
  and reactive hypoglycemia, 80
  and sugar consumption, 7, 80
blood sugar. *See also*
  hyperglycemia; hypoglycemia;
  hypoglycemia, reactive
  regulation of, 47–48
  variations in level of, *51*
bread. *See* grains
breakfast, *143*
  effect of, on blood sugar, 138–43
  and lack of morning appetite,
  146–49
  making, a priority, 144–49

brown rice, 59, *95,* 101, 123. *See
    also* grains
    flour, 37, 124
    syrup, 125, 127
brown sugar, 26, 109
bulimia, 79

candy, manufacture of, 13
cane sugar (sucrose), 42. *See also*
    sugarcane cultivation
carbohydrates, 39
    content of certain foods, *45*
    foods with good sugar, 21
    kinds of, 39–44, *44*
    need for, 44–46
    and proteins, 139–42
cardiovascular diseases, 64
Carton, Dr. Paul, 17–19
cellulitis, 66
cellulose, 43–44
cereal. *See* grains
China, and history of sugarcane
    cultivation, 12
coconut, *95*
    flour, 37, *94,* 124
    sugar, 125, 127
confectioners' sugar/syrup, 27
consumption of refined sugar,
    7–19, *8*
cooking and glycemic index, 101
corn syrup, 27
Crusades, effect of, on sugar's use, 13

dairy products, inability to digest,
    42

date syrup, 125, 126
deficiencies of nutrients, 57–60,
    58, 59
dehydration, 151–54, *153*
dependency on refined sugar,
    83–86
dextrose (fruit sugar), 28, 40
diabetes, 67–71
    elimination of bad sugars, 118
    proteins, influence of, on, 141
disaccharides, 41–42, *44*
diseases caused by bad sugars,
    118–19
    acidification, 60–62, *61*
    diabetes, 67–71
    diseases caused by colloidal
        toxins, 64–65
    obesity, 65–66
    poisoning of body, 62–64
    starvation, 57–60
disorders caused by reactive
    hypoglycemia, 79–86
drinks with refined sugar, 111

elimination of bad sugars, 115–20
energy, low, causes of, 150–51
    acid-alkaline imbalance,
        154–57
    dehydration, 151–54, *153*
    sedentary lifestyle, 157–59
environmental impact of sugar
    production, 17
enzymes, 151
exercise
    dehydration and, 152

and drawing from body's
reserves, 158–59

fake foods, 4–6
fast vs. slow sugars, 132–36
flour. *See* grains
food cravings and diabetes, 68
food in pounds consumed by
average American, *8*
foods high in refined sugar,
109–12, *130–31*
foods with hidden sugars, 112–13
fructose (fruit sugar), 28, 40
fruits, 21
and glycemic index, *94, 95, 96,*
98–99
with good sugars, 123
sugar content of, 6
fuel, sugar as, 1

galactose, 40
genetic engineering of sugar beets.
See sugar beets
glucose, 27, 40, 41
conversion of, in hyperglycemia,
53
toxic acids, effect on, 62
gluten sensitivity, *36,* 134
flour options for, 37–38
glycemia, 47–48. *See also*
hyperglycemia; hypoglycemia;
hypoglycemia, reactive
glycemic index
bad sugars and, 102–4
determining, 92–93

differences in foods, 98–102
and fast vs. slow sugars, 132, 134
ranking foods, 93–98, *94, 95,*
96, 103
and weight gain, 104–5
glycosuria (sugar in urine), 7
government efforts to reduce bad
sugars, 160
grains, 21. *See also* brown rice
cereal grains, puffed, and
glycemic index, 102
flour, foods high in refined
white, 114–15
flour, production of, 32–34
flour, white, reason to consume,
119
flours, sugar in, 114
flours, wheat, 34–35, *36*
flours other than wheat, 37–38
and glycemic index, *94, 95, 96,* 99
with good sugars, 123–25,
130–31
mineral content of, *59*
refined, 113–14
refinement of, 22, *30,* 30–32
vitamin content of flours, *58*
grape cure, 7
grape sugar, 40
Greece, and history of sugarcane
cultivation, 11

hidden sugars, foods with, 112–13
high-fructose corn syrup, 27
honey, 21
sugar content of, 6

hyperglycemia, 48–50, 51, *51,*
    52–53, *53*
  diabetic hyperglycemic crisis, 70
  proteins, influence of, on, 141
hypoglycemia, 50–51, 53–56, *55.*
    See also hypoglycemia,
    reactive
  proteins, influence of, on, 141
hypoglycemia, reactive, 72–86, *74*
  diet test for, 87–89
  elimination, need for, 118
  symptoms test for, 89–92

ice cream, 27, *96,* 110, *130*
India, and history of sugarcane
    cultivation, 10–12
infection and diabetes, 69
insulin. *See also* pancreas, role of
  and glycemic index, 93
  and obesity, 66
invert sugar, 27

ketoacidosis, 68–69

lactase deficiency, 42
lactose (milk sugar), 41
legumes, 21
levulose, 40
liquid sugar, 27
liver weakness, 64
low energy, causes of, 150–51
  dehydration, 151–54, *153*

maltose (malt sugar), 41, *44,* 125,
    127, *130*

maple syrup, 55, 125, *130*
mental disorders and reactive
    hypoglycemia, 81–86
milk sugar (lactose), 41–42
mineral content
  of different sugars, *24*
  of grains, *59*
molasses, 125, 126, *130*
  dark, value of, 23, 24
  table, 28
monosaccharides, 40–41, *44*

Napoleon's blockade, as
    cause of increase in sugar
    consumption, 15–19
New World, sugarcane plantations
    in, 13–14
nut allergies, coconut flour
    for, 37

obesity, 65–66
  and glycemic index, 104–5
organic sugar, 25–26

pancreas, role of. *See also* insulin
  in diabetes, 67, 70
  in reactive hypoglycemia,
    72–86, *74,* 118
  in regulating blood sugar, 52–53,
    53, 55, *55,* 140–41, 147
pasta. *See* grains
peanuts, 21
pear concentrate, 125, 126
Persia, and history of sugarcane
    cultivation, 12–13

plant starch, 43
polysaccharides, 42–43, *44*
potatoes, 21
profit, as motive for
    manufacture of fake foods, 5
proteins, adding, 137–43, *143*
psychological reasons for eating
    bad sugars, 120–21
"pure" sugar, definition of, 23

refined sugar. *See also* sugar,
    bad
    consumption of, 7–19
    foods high in, 109–12
    health, impact on, 17
    history of, 4–19
    kinds of, 25–29, 108–9
    medical uses for, 12
    metabolization of, 6–7
    use of, in food, 14–15
    replacing bad sugars with good
        sugars, 128–31, *130–31*
respiratory ailments, 64–65
rice. *See* brown rice; grains
rock candy, 13, 28

sclerosis, 69
skin disorders, 65, 70
slavery and sugarcane
    plantations, 14
slow vs. fast sugars, 132–36
soy, 21, 123
    components of, 5
sports. *See* exercise
standard menu, 115–17

starches, 42–43
    and glycemic index, 100–101
    starchy foods with good sugars,
        123
stevia, 127–28
"stone honey," 12
sucrose, 5, 42
sugar, bad. *See also* refined sugar
    and adulteration of food, 22
    composition of, *24*
    excessive desire for, 77–79
    extraction of, 22–24
    government efforts to reduce
        bad sugars, 160
    harmful effects of, 3
    hidden sugars, foods with,
        112–13
    identifying and eliminating,
        108–21
    psychological reasons for eating,
        120–21
    replacing, with good sugars,
        128–31, *130–31*
sugar, good, 25. *See also* molasses,
    dark, value of
    composition of, *24*
    in foods, 20–21, 123–25
    as fuel, 1
    kinds of, 25–29
    natural sweeteners, 125–28
    reasons for eating, 122
    replacing bad sugars with,
        128–31, *130–31*
sugar, raw, 23, 25–26
    composition of, *24*

sugar beets
    extraction process for, 23
    genetic engineering of, 17
    as source of sugar, 15–16, 42
sugarcane cultivation, 9–16,
    22–23
sugars, fast vs. slow, 132–36
sweeteners
    natural, 125–28, *130–31*
    synthetic, 29, 111–12,
        130–31

thirst and diabetes, 68. *See also*
    dehydration
thyroid gland and regulation
    of blood sugar, 55, *55*
turbinado sugar, 26

urine and diabetes, 68

vegetables, 21
    with good sugar, 123
    sugar content of, 6
vitamin content
    of different sugars, *24*
    of grains, 59

water. *See* dehydration
weight gain. *See* obesity
whey powder, 42
white sugar. *See* refined sugar;
    sugar, bad
whole sugar. *See* sugar, good

xylitol, 28

BOOKS OF RELATED INTEREST

The Acid-Alkaline Diet for Optimum Health
Restore Your Health by Creating pH Balance in Your Diet
by Christopher Vasey, N.D.

Freedom from Constipation
Natural Remedies for Digestive Health
by Christopher Vasey, N.D.

Liver Detox
Cleansing through Diet, Herbs, and Massage
by Christopher Vasey, N.D.

Natural Remedies for Inflammation
by Christopher Vasey, N.D.

Natural Antibiotics and Antivirals
18 Infection-Fighting Herbs and Essential Oils
by Christopher Vasey, N.D.

Natural Compresses and Poultices
Safe and Simple Folk Medicine Treatments
for 70 Common Conditions
by Christopher Vasey, N.D.

Healing the Thyroid with Ayurveda
Natural Treatments for Hashimoto's,
Hypothyroidism, and Hyperthyroidism
by Marianne Teitelbaum, D.C.
Foreword by Anjali Grover, M.D.

Primal Body, Primal Mind
Beyond Paleo for Total Health and a Longer Life
by Nora Gedgaudas, CNS, NTP, BCHN

INNER TRADITIONS • BEAR & COMPANY
P.O. Box 388 • Rochester, VT 05767
1-800-246-8648
www.InnerTraditions.com

Or contact your local bookseller